DATE DUE

FEB 1 8 1994	
MAR 2 8 1994	
JAN 1 6 1997	
MAR 2 4 1998	
OCT 2 7 1998	
NOV 1 9 1998	
JUN 1 8 1999	
JUN 1 8 1999	
OCT 4 1999	
FEB 2 4 2000	
MAY 2 3 2000	
NOV 2 1 2001	

BRODART   Cat. No. 23-221

Children's Stress and Coping

PERSPECTIVES ON MARRIAGE AND THE FAMILY
Bert N. Adams and David M. Klein, *Editors*

WIFE BATTERING: A SYSTEMS THEORY APPROACH
Jean Giles-Sim

COMMUTER MARRIAGE: A STUDY OF WORK AND FAMILY
Naomi Gerstel and Harriet Gross

HELPING THE ELDERLY: THE COMPLEMENTARY ROLES
OF INFORMAL NETWORKS AND FORMAL SYSTEMS
Eugene Litwak

REMARRIAGE AND STEPPARENTING:
CURRENT RESEARCH AND THEORY
Kay Palsey and Marilyn Ihinger-Tallman (Eds.)

FEMINISM. CHILDREN, AND THE NEW FAMILIES
Sanford M. Dornbusch and Myta F. Strober (Eds.)

DYNAMICS OF FAMILY DEVELOPMENT:
A THEORETICAL PERSPECTIVE
James M. White

PORTRAIT OF DIVORCE:
ADJUSTMENT TO MARITAL BREAKDOWN
Gay C. Kitson with William M. Holmes

WOMEN AND FAMILIES: FEMINIST RECONSTRUCTIONS
Kristine M. Baber and Katherine R. Allen

CHILDREN'S STRESS AND COPING:
A FAMILY PERSPECTIVE
Elaine Shaw Sorensen

Children's Stress and Coping

A Family Perspective

ELAINE SHAW SORENSEN

THE GUILFORD PRESS

New York   London

© 1993 The Guilford Press
A Division of Guilford Publications, Inc.
72 Spring Street, New York, NY 10012

Printed in the United States of America

This book is printed on acid-free paper.

Last digit is print number: 9 8 7 6 5 4 3 2 1

Library of Congress Cataloging-in-Publication Data

Sorensen, Elaine Shaw.
    Children's stress and coping : a family perspective / Elaine Shaw
Sorensen.
        p.   cm. —(Perspectives on marriage and the family)
    Includes bibliographical references and index.
    ISBN 0-89862-084-8
    1. Stress in children.   2. Adjustment (Psychology) in children.
I. Title.   II. Series.
    [DNLM: 1. Adaptation, Psychological—in infancy & childhood.
2. Family—psychology.   3. Stress, Psychological—in infancy &
childhood.   WS 350 S713c]
BF723.S75S67   1993
155.4'18—dc20
DNLM/DLC
for Library of Congress   92-48859
                                                              CIP

For Rulon and Jean,
Brian, Chad, Johanna,
. . . and Todd

The terms "stress" and "coping" have almost become clichés in professional and popular literature. We seem to encounter stress-events lists and stress-management advice at every turn, from the social science library to the grocery check-out. Unfortunately, however, stress remains a daily, universal reality, and effective responses continue to be as elusive as ever. Stress affects each member of the family, as well as the entire family unit. Despite increasing interest in stress–coping research among adults and families, little is known about how stress is actually perceived by children in the setting of their own families.

My interest in stress–coping phenomena began in a graduate introductory course in stress management. As the course progressed and I practiced the prescribed techniques, I found amazingly little to associate with my own daily life. Sources of stress in adults, families, and children have largely been identified as particular life events, traumatic situations, or demands for change. And stress management programs have primarily been directed toward the promotion of relaxation techniques. Extensive study has related stress to illness and maladaptation. But few investigations have been directed toward the proportion of study populations that remains healthy or seems able to avoid or overcome maladaptive effects of stress. Peck (1978) proposes that although science has been able to identify determinants of illness and cure, it has not been able to do so for the origins of resistance and health:

> We know very well why people become . . . ill. What we don't understand is why people survive the traumas of their lives as well as they do. . . . All we can say is that there is a force, the mechanics of which we do not fully understand, that seems to operate routinely in most people to protect and to foster their . . . health even under the most adverse conditions. . . . We know a great deal more about the causes of physical disease than we do about the causes of physical health. (pp. 237–239)

There have been few studies of how healthy people cope with the ordinary stress of daily life. Currently, some researchers are assessing adult stress and coping in day-to-day life. However, there has been little exploration of stress and coping processes in the daily lives of children, particularly from the holistic perspective of the family.

As a mother, I have found few professional applications which I could imagine being relevant for my own children. I have been struck by the need to see the world of children from the child's own viewpoint. This point came in clearly one evening in a restaurant as I dined with my four children. As I repeated the usual litany from the children's menu to my 5-year-old daughter—grilled cheese sandwich, hot dog, spaghetti (the children's menu is the same, no matter what the restaurant)—she interrupted indignantly, "This time I'm ordering from the *human* menu!"

From my own children, and from the children for whom I have cared as a nurse in clinical practice, I have learned that children live in a unique culture that most of us have forgotten; that children, if given a chance, can and will readily articulate the joys and vicissitudes of their daily life. Further, children are capable of sharing insights into their own needs and responses.

The difficulty in studying children's stress and coping within the family realm has been potentiated by inadequacies in conceptual frameworks and by methodological complexities, such as recognizing and studying appropriate informants, or measuring aggregate and individual data. Further, issues of stress–coping phenomena have most often reflected marital, child-rearing, or life-transition challenges reported by adults. Subjective data from the child's view of family life are sparse. There is a need for multidisciplinary collaboration and for merging theoretical philosophies and methodologies that accommodate variables from the viewpoints of individual and aggregate, child and parent, pathology and health.

The purpose of this work is to explore issues in the study of stress–coping phenomena, and to identify and describe daily stressors and coping responses as actually experienced and reported by school-age children.

Chapter One reviews various perspectives for the study of stress-coping phenomena. Among the perspectives described are the: (1) individual perspective on individuals, (2) family perspective on families, (3) adult perspective on children, (4) child perspective on children, and (5) family perspective on children. Traditional definitions of stress and coping variables are then described, which largely reflect an individual perspective on individuals. The works reviewed in Chapter

One have set the traditional course for definition of concepts and approaches to study. Implications for current child and family study are offered.

In Chapter Two, the foundation of the individual's perspective is carried further into family study, reflecting a family perspective on families. The chapter deals largely with theoretical viewpoints, exploring traditional theoretical frameworks in family and stress–coping study. I then suggest an integrated approach to family stress–coping theory, combining concepts and methods from a classic family stress-crisis theory and a cognitive–transactional stess–coping model. General areas in family stress research are then reviewed, with critique pointing to specific needs related to the study of children within the family.

Concepts of stess–coping phenomena specifically among children are reviewed in Chapter Three, reflecting the children's perspective on children. Concepts of stress, coping, appraisal, and mediating variables and interventions are discussed as they appear in research literature about children. Implications for theory and methods are explored.

Chapter Four offers a report of my own study of daily stressors, coping responses, and mediating resources as actually experienced and reported by a group of 42 healthy school-age children. Data were drawn from semistructured daily journals kept by children and parents over a period of 6 weeks. Content analysis resulted in taxonomies of daily stressors, coping responses, and coping resources, with comparisons of their frequencies among parents, boys, and girls. Such taxonomies are an attempt to organize the rich data from children, in order to provide foundations for future research and valid instrument development. Direct comparison of child and parent diaries also revealed specific themes reflecting high and low scores on parents' ability to take the perspective of the children in reporting daily stess–coping phenomena.

Such data offer insights into a family perspective of children's daily stess–coping experiences and allow a descriptive exploration of relationships among stress, coping, and resource themes.

Children's diaries included the option of daily colored drawings. The value of children's spontaneous art work as enriching, qualitative, descriptive data is described in Chapter Five. Drawings enhanced the diary entries, and offered insights into the child's view of family phenomena. A few actual drawings are shared. Though some of the detail and richness of the original colored drawings are lost in their black-and-white presentation here, the whole picture of children's perceptions would be incomplete without them.

Chapter Six reviews the meaning for research and clinical practice of both the literature analyses of Chapters One through Three, and the actual data reported in Chapters Four and Five. Epistemological viewpoints are explored, as well as needs in empirical research and clinical practice among children.

Two pervading themes throughout all chapters are the need for refinement of methods and for increased multidisciplinary approaches to study. Literature is reviewed in the disciplines of sociology, psychology, family studies, nursing, medicine, art therapy, child development, and others. Needless to say I am not an expert in so many fields and the review is not exhaustive. However, while surveying such vast and varied works, I was struck by both overlap and gaps in the areas of concept definition, theory development, and valid clinical application related to families and children. The extent of the contributions of disciplines to the study of stress and coping is daunting. We now need to begin to learn each other's languages, integrate, and validly test our combined knowledge.

This book offers a critical review of current scholarship related to children and families, and provides the actual results of a particular study of children. Taking such an approach—making bold critiques and suggestions related to the theories, methods, and practice of others, while reporting on an original empirical study that does not adequately address all the issues raised—exposes the author to a risk. I take that risk, acknowledging that my own study, reported in Chapters Four and Five, does not respond to all issues, concerns, and needs described in Chapters One through Three and Six. However, I offer the work as an attempt to begin to see and respond to the subjective view of families, particularly the child's viewpoint within the family.

ACKNOWLEDGMENTS

To Jerry Braza, Patrick Walsh, Onie Grosshans, John Wolfer, and Beryl Peters for nurturing the seed of this work, and to June Leifson, Lynn Callister, and Carolyn Melby, for encouraging its growth.

To Alana Knutson for offering a fresh critical view of tired data.

To Roger Flick, Brenda Evans, and Virginia Watson at the Harold B. Lee Library at Brigham Young University for expert support and interest.

To David Klein, Bert Adams, Sharon Panulla, Susan Marples, and Anna Brackett for patience and encouragement.

Especially, to David Klein for stretching my thinking, and extending intellectual connections that continue to enrich my work.

To Guilford Publications and the National Council on Family Relations for according me the honor of the Student/New Professional Book Award, which cultivated the seed to full growth.

Finally, to the children and parents of this study, who willingly shared their daily lives.

C O N T E N T S

Children's Stress and Coping

Perspectives for Study: Traditional Approaches to Stress and Coping

Stress affects every system within the human organism, as well as every human social system, including the family. Cultural changes exert escalating pressures on modern families, requiring children to endure stressors unknown to previous generations. Helping children and families to cope successfully with life trauma and daily life stress is of increasing interest to nurses, social scientists, and family therapists. It is the purpose of this book to explore the psychosocial stressors and coping responses of daily life from the viewpoint of school-age children. The work views the child in the context of the family, rather than as an individual in a clinical setting, and highlights the value of the child as an informant in family research.

The concepts of stress and coping, as they apply to family research and therapy, emerge from the evolution of many biological and psychosocial pursuits. Scientific interest in this body of knowledge has proliferated in recent years, due partially to its universal relevance. Professional reports and public literature offer an abundance of theoretical, methodological, and empirical explorations of stress and coping (see Appley & Trumbull, 1986; Boss, 1988; Field, McCabe, & Schneiderman, 1988; Garmezy & Rutter, 1983; Kasl & Cooper, 1987; Lazarus & Folkman, 1984; McCubbin & Figley, 1983; McCubbin, Sussman, & Patterson, 1983; Monat & Lazarus, 1991).

A research study of stress–coping phenomena among school-age children will be reported later in the book. This chapter will review perspectives, traditional conceptual definitions, and research approaches, providing a historical foundation in concept development, context, and direction for the study to be reported.

PERSPECTIVES AND CONCEPTUAL MAPS FOR STUDY

Before such a review, it is important to understand both the perspectives and analytical matrix by which concepts are examined. First, the study of stress experiences among individuals and families has been approached from several important perspectives. Although theorists and researchers often approach concepts from assumed viewpoints or contexts, it is important to recognize that there may be several epistemological perspectives. The idea of "perspective" here may have three related meanings: (1) the point of view that is represented, (2) the unit of analysis, and (3) the types of explanatory factors that are involved. Some examples of the viewpoints for study of stress–coping phenomena among families are listed below:

1. *An individual perspective on individuals.* This viewpoint defines stress–coping phenomena from the perspective of the individual's experience that may or may not include related interactions with other individuals or groups, such as the family. The work of Lazarus and Folkman (1984) is probably the best example of this perspective.

2. *An individual perspective on families.* This viewpoint reveals the experience of an individual in relation to interaction with family members and situations. Some of the work on stress management seems to emerge from this point of view, where interventions are aimed at individuals, with family factors included as antecedent or outcome variables.

3. *A family perspective on families.* This type of framework examines the interpersonal stressors and/or coping strategies and styles that are characteristic of the entire group called "family." Examples among the works of McCubbin and colleagues (McCubbin & Figley, 1983; McCubbin, Sussman, & Patterson, 1983) use a viewpoint of stress perceptions and coping styles as experienced by the entire family unit. Indeed, most theoretical and empirical efforts in family studies would probably fall into this category.

4. *A situational perspective on individuals, families, or children.* This more distal approach studies stress–coping phenomena within conceptual, social, or environmental contexts as they relate to the individual or family unit. It would provide a "wider" (social, biological, demographic, extra-familial, social systems, etc.) viewpoint on family members or units. Examples include the numerous demographic analyses of family phenomena or studies from cultural, legal–political, educational, medical, or other institutional systems. Other examples are those works that

focus on particular stressor events or life transitions (i.e., the advent of parenting, retirement, or elder-care, or illness, bereavement, etc.) and subsequent individual or family responses. Distal social and environmental contexts related specifically to children might include the neighborhood–peer–friend culture, characteristics or perceptions of the school environment, occupational patterns of parents, or even influences of larger economic or political situations.

5. *An individual (adult) perspective on children.* This viewpoint represents the traditional study of stress–coping phenomena in children, which has devised instruments and drawn conclusions about children based on revised adult-framed knowledge. Examples include the life-events lists and stress-management interventions for children that are adapted from the adult versions. Other examples include works where adults, such as parents, teachers, or clinicians serve as informants about children.

6. *A child perspective on children and/or families.* A few studies have attempted to describe stress–coping phenomena from the viewpoint of children themselves. Yamamoto, Soliman, Parsons, and Davies's (1987) rankings of stressors by children, and the use of children's subjective responses by investigators such as Ryan (1988), Sorensen (1990, 1991), and Walker (1986) provide examples.

7. *A family perspective on children.* This type of framework explores the effects of proximal family phenomena on the responses of individual family members. The study of children from the viewpoint of the individual family unit is a fairly rare, but important, approach to understanding children and families. Children are the analytical units, while family variables become proximal, contextual antecedents and/or consequences. A family perspective on children might also focus on interpersonal stressors and coping responses for familial subgroups, such as parent–child dyads, or child sibling groups.

This list is not exhaustive and represents only explanatory viewpoints for study, not ways of knowing based on philosophy of science. Indeed, each perspective mentioned might be approached from a number of epistemological philosophies, such as positivistic, phenomenological, and feminist, to name a few.

Larzelere and Klein (1987) described a similar matrix adapted from Levinger (1977) for generating research questions and explaining methodological approaches. Along two axes of antecedent variables and consequent variables, their matrix listed the following units of analysis: individual, dyad, nuclear family, extended family, situation, and society. For emphasis, I have added the unit of children, which should fall under the unit of "individual," in the study to be described. Walker (1985) also argued that the interdependent levels of individual, dyad, family group, social network, community, and culture/history must be accommodated in the development of family stress theory.

The study to be described later in this book (Chapter 4) assumes *a family perspective on children* (perspective 7). However, the direct perspective of children on themselves (perspective 6) is also of primary importance for the validity of the study. In addition, to a limited extent, the viewpoints of other individuals (parents and siblings) (perspective 5) are provided.

The preceding list of approaches also applies to the study of many phenomena other than stress and coping. Indeed, Larzelere and Klein's (1987) matrix was proposed generically as a framework for generating and clarifying any questions, concepts, and propositions in family study. Most research in family studies would claim to fit into category 3 — "a family perspective on families" — and theorists and researchers, however unintentionally, often see that viewpoint as the only way to study every topic relevant to studies of families. Such a limited approach to context is unfortunately common in social science research.

Acknowledging the viewpoint of a study is important because it influences both data sources and assumptions in analysis. There is some controversy about which data source best represents the assumed point of view. For example, if one represents the viewpoint of the child, it seems reasonable to argue that data ought to originate from the child at the cultural and developmental level of the child, rather than from an adult report.

Further, it seems reasonable to expect that a "family perspective" would draw data from several, if not all, family members. Unfortunately, few instruments have been developed to accommodate either the point of view of young children or the complexity of multiple informants.

Recognition of perspective, or point of view represented, is only one aspect of study in a complex conceptual scheme. Thus, to trace a conceptual map of stress–coping phenomena in children and families can be a complex epistemological task. The image becomes less that of a map, with a linear route to a specific conceptual destination, but rather that of a multidimensional matrix, with attempts to untangle and reweave conceptual threads.

Primary among the tangled yarns is the definition of terms. The term "stress" has been used to refer to physiological, psychological, and social demands, each with long continua of perception and severity. The importance of physiological factors in stress and health, usually as dependent variables, is well recognized in clinical study. However, the larger body of this work will focus on psychosocial stressors and responses. The concept of coping as a response to stressors includes factors of perception or appraisal, as well as individual and environmental resources.

A contrasting thread lies in units of observation. Units of observation include individuals (children and adults) and social groups (nonfamilial and familial). Nonfamilial groups could include occupational groups or groups brought together by particular stressful events, such as prisoners of war or inpatient groups. This work will not address nonfamilial groups.

Another knotty issue is that of "family." Units of analysis in family research have included individuals and groups, including the marital couple, parent–child dyads, and sibling groups. Stress has been examined within families, upon families, and interactionally within and upon various individual family members. Other factors, such as stressed relationships (not simply stressed persons) or family variables as either antecedent or dependent variables in stress–coping phenomena, further compound the issues of the matrix. In this study the "family" studied was the traditional parents-with-minor-children nuclear household.

The other major concept relevant to this study is that of "children." While some may use the term "children" broadly according to a familial relationship—that is, one who is chronologically subordinate to a parent regardless of age—this work assumes the traditional developmental prima facie view of the child as the minor offspring within a family. Acknowledging some references to preschool, adolescent, or even to adult children, the study to be reported may only be validly generalized to school-age children.

As a historical background for clarification, rationale, and "reweaving" of the study to be reported herein, this chapter will review traditional conceptual issues in stress and coping and will explore foundation works that emphasized adult individuals as the unit of analysis, with brief references to related works on children and families. This chapter will also discuss traditional definitions of stress and coping, the nature of the problems studied, and implications for research about children and families.

TRADITIONAL STRESS-COPING DEFINITIONS AND INTERPRETATIONS

Stress

The first major obstacle in conducting an inquiry into stress–coping phenomena has been the absence of an adequate, generally accepted definition of stress. Historically, several interpretations have been used. As in other areas of early social research, terms and methods were borrowed from the physical sciences. Hence, early definitions included such concepts as "forces, stress, cause and effect, resistance, dynamics, and determinism" (Sorensen, 1986, p. 5). Cannon (1932) described stress as a disturbance of homeostasis under extreme internal or external environmental conditions, and proposed that the degree of stress might be measured.

Selye (1974) defined stress as the "nonspecific response of the body to any demand made upon it" (p. 14). He further recognized the concept of "eustress," as "good" stress that does not provoke maladaptive responses. Selye's interpretation of stress as a fairly predictable constellation of psychophysiological responses to noxious stimuli called stressors, described in his General Adaptation Syndrome (Selye, 1956), significantly influenced modern stress–coping research. Subsequent definitions of stress, following Selye's orientation, include the following:

1. The physical or mental effect or disturbance of, or interference with, any of the body's automatic biological processes (Stephan, 1971)
2. A psychophysiological arousal which, if prolonged, can fatigue, damage, or lead to disease in the organism (Girdano & Everly, 1979)
3. A condition in which a discrepancy exists between the demands, loss, threatened loss, or life events and the individual's capacity to respond, thus threatening conditions essential to health (Caplan, 1976)
4. The result of unsuccessful coping (Swogger, 1981)

Obviously, there has been some ambiguity in defining stress as to whether it refers to the stimulus (some call this the stressor), to an intervening process, or to the resultant maladaptive factor in health and illness. Mason (1975) noted that "the term 'stress' has been used variously to refer to 'stimulus' by some workers, 'responses' by some workers, 'interaction' by others, and more comprehensive combinations of the above factors by still other workers" (p. 29). Rutter (1983) observed that "stress seems to apply equally to a form of stimulus (or stressor), a force requiring change of adaptation (strain), a mental state (distress), and a form of bodily reaction or response (that is, Selye's general adaptation syndrome of stress)" (p. 1). However, Lazarus (1966) asserted that stress is not "stimulus, responses, or intervening variables, but rather a collective term for an area of study" (p. 27).

Monat and Lazarus (1991) identified three major types of stress: systemic or physiological, psychological, and social. Definitions and relationships among these types of stress are integrally entangled. For example, perceived psychological or social stressors are well known to cause or exacerbate physiological stress. Lazarus and associates (Lazarus & Folkman, 1984; Monat & Lazarus, 1991) proposed a process approach to the definition of stress as a relationship between the person, tissue system, or social system and the environment that is appraised by the individual, family, or other social system as taxing or exceeding resources and endangering well-being.

Because it is difficult to define stress scientifically, some have suggested that the term "stress" be abandoned in scientific inquiry, while others argue for the use of the term as a generic, collective label for a complex, interdisciplinary area of interest. Mullan (1983) suggested the following:

> I would advocate that the word "stress" be stricken from our vocabulary as soon as possible. There is no consensus among scholars about its exact referent — and it carries an unfortunate amount of conceptual baggage. It is time in our theorizing to avoid the highly-charged language which equates environmental demands, such as events and transitions, with significant personal and familial change, and then significant change with distress or disorganization. This suggestion is especially important when we are discussing events and transitions for which we have little solid evidence about their actual difficulty for individuals or families.

Although I agree with the difficulties pointed out by Mullan, I would hesitate to discard the term "stress," since science is yet unable to offer a better, more precise term. The concept of stress seems to encompass a general body of study. In apparent efforts to impose more concrete parameters, many have attempted to define stress in terms of particular life events.

Stress Events

With the advent of stress-events scales, stress came to be viewed as a state provoked by particular life-change situations, with additive implications. The widely used stress-events scale of Holmes and Rahe (1967), which listed several life events and rated and ranked them according to a particular cumulative stress score, was thought to correlate with illness onset. Coddington (1972) developed a similar measure for life-stress events among children of various age groups.

In attempts to demonstrate family stress, some have correlated parent and child stress-events scores, though a simple examination of the scales reveals the lists to be highly similar, with scales for children developed from the viewpoint of adults' or parents' life events, without validation by children themselves. Furthermore, the reverberating effects of individual life events upon other family members has not been addressed from the context of major-life-events theory. Although some scales for family life events have been developed (McCubbin, Patterson, & Wilson, 1983), theoretical and methodological questions of what constitutes and who interprets "family life events" are still unanswered.

Paykel (1974) added to stress-events theory the framework of life's entrances and exits, and underscored the clinical significance of perception of events. Hetherington (1984) studied these concepts from the viewpoint of compounding events, for example, demonstrating that children adjust more effectively to a life stress such as divorce when the situation is not complicated by many other more minor stressors. McCubbin and associates (McCubbin & McCubbin, 1987; McCubbin, Patterson, & Wilson, 1983) further conceptualized the idea of the accumulation or "pileup" of stressors in families. Indeed, the very validity of scores on Holmes and Rahe's (1967) life-events scale is dependent upon an accumulation of events over a relatively short period of time.

Life-change events became the most dominant measure of stress in numerous correlation studies relating stress-events scores to illness. Stress was viewed as the culmination of environmental change (Johnson, 1986). Paykel (1974) and Miller (1981) observed that some stress events were negative, in the sense that they were undesirable, while others were positive and thus socially or individually desired. They argued that it was perception, required adaptation, and the factor of *change* that precipitated individual stress. Burr (1973) also added the dimension of change to his modification of Hill's (1949) family stress theory.

However, Weinberg, and Richardson (1981) cited several studies indicating that "it is not change per se but undesirable or negative change that is stressful" (p. 686) and that what is stressful about life events are more detailed characteristics of the events themselves and the perceptions of the individual. Ryan (1988) cautioned against the use of life-events scales because (1) they do not distinguish between desirable or undesirable change, and (2) they do not allow for appraisal of the stressfulness of particular stress events.

Recent analysis invokes increasing caution in the use of life events as measures for stress. Life events are portrayed as single events of trauma, such as death or illness of a family member, divorce, natural disaster, or war, or as normal role transitions, such as first births, child rearing, or retirement. Mullan (1983) warned against the uncritical acceptance of the life-events framework with its illusive ease in producing quantifiable stress scores and its pervasive influence in models for family stress. He pointed out several significant empirical and methodological problems in the wholesale acceptance of life-events theory, including subjects' inaccurate and selective recall of events, confounding of events with psychological and physiological symptoms they purport to predict, and ineffective checklists which produce less reliable data than other techniques, such as personal interview.

Lazarus and Folkman (1984) discussed extensively the apparent inadequacy and "atheoretical" nature of life-events theory as the only definition or measure of stress:

> A striking feature of stress research is the overwhelming concern with . . . life events. . . .
>
> There are major defects in the assumptions underlying the life events approach that make it inadequate as the sole metric of stress. The first assumption is that the life events approach to stress measurement assumes that change alone is stressful. . . .
>
> A second assumption is that life events must be major, that is, have profound adaptational consequence of sufficient magnitude to impair health. Although this thinking seems reasonable . . . it is incomplete in important ways. Simply knowing that life events have occurred does not permit us to grasp their individual meanings—what they do to the appraised person–environment relationship—and how they are responded to in the present on a day-to-day basis. . . .
>
> A third assumption is that psychological stress is a major factor in illness. . . .
>
> The practical problem that flows from the limits and defects in these assumptions is that the relationship between life events indices and health outcomes is small and accounts for only a small proportion of the variance in health outcomes. . . . Thus, life events have little practical significance in the prediction of health outcomes, even though such prediction is the prime reason for using life-events indices. (pp. 309–310)

In observing adult roles and responses to life stresses, Pearlin (1991) proposed the idea of scheduled and nonscheduled events, termed "life strains." He divided strains into three major categories that may elicit emotional distress. These include (1) the daily, enduring "slow-to-change" problems; (2) predictable, regular events of the life cycle, such as marriage, childbirth, or retirement; and (3) unscheduled, usually undesirable, eruptive events, such as illness, divorce, or premature death of a loved one. Though such a framework resembles the work of some family scientists, Pearlin's description includes neither a family context nor children beyond their antecedent effects on the development of the individual adult.

Although the concept of major life events, or change, as a definition of stress is attracting increasing scrutiny and criticism, the idea of stress as an event rather than a process continues to influence the direction of research. This is evident to some extent in the recent interest in the study of minor events or "hassles" as sources of stress.

Daily Hassles

Lazarus and Folkman (1984) pointed to studies that found daily stressors over time, or hassles, "far superior" to life events in the prediction of psychological or physiological variables (DeLongis, Coyne, Dakof, Folkman, & Lazarus, 1982; Kanner, Coyne, Schaefer, & Lazarus, 1981) and affirmed the need for replication of such inquiries. To define stress as a major life event such as bereavement, divorce, or chronic illness is to limit the concept and to overlook a large constellation of factors that affect health and adaptation. Ordinary daily life is filled with what some term "hassles": time constraints, loneliness, losing a favorite possession, family arguments, feeling left out of friends' activities, or getting a bad grade. These less dramatic situations are far more common, more affected by cognitive appraisal, more conducive to prevention or treatment, more important in adaptation, and appear to be better predictors of health than major life events (Lazarus & Folkman, 1984).

Kanner and colleagues (1981) developed a list of hassles for adults, and Kanner, Feldman, Weinberger, and Ford (1991) have begun the work with such variables among children. Crnic and associates have begun to study daily hassles in relation to parenting. One study (Crnic & Greenberg, 1990) reported mothers' perceptions of daily hassles related to care of their 5-year-old children to be more predictive of several aspects of parental satisfaction and family functioning than major life stresses. Another study (Crnic & Booth, 1991) reported that hassles increased as children's ages increased, and that social support effectively moderated hassles. With the exception of recent measures that include family "strains" (McCubbin, Patterson, & Wilson, 1983), less is known about the significance of hassles from the viewpoint of an entire family unit, either within or outside the family–home environment.

The study of hassles promises to open the arena for a broader understanding of the dimensions of stress as events. However, if we acknowledge that the concept of stress includes facets beyond life events, major or minor, we must recognize other means to measure stress. Social scientists continue to struggle with this issue.

Other Measures of Stress

One of the most interesting evidences of the difficulty of arriving at a universally acceptable definition of stress is the association of stress with particular personality characteristics. Characteristics such as anxiety, fear, or vulnerability have been studied as both mediating variables in the stress–coping process and as conceptual or operational definitions of stress itself.

Since Spielberger's (1966) empirical assessment of trait anxiety, that concept became frequently and conveniently interpreted as a measure for stress. In the past, anxiety was interpreted by some as a drive force in pathological adaptation to stress (Lazarus, 1981). Several studies presented stress and anxiety as operationally synonymous (Auerbach, Martelli, & Mercuri, 1983; LaMontagne, Mason, & Hepworth, 1985).

Another common interpretation of stress has been as Type A behavior patterns, characterized by aggressiveness, competitiveness, a sense of time urgency, and free-floating anger, first described by Friedman and Rosenman (1974). A similar syndrome has been described among children and correlated with health indicators (Bishop, Hailey, & Anderson, 1987; Eagleston et al., 1986; Thoresen, Eagleston, Kirmil-Gray, & Bracke, 1985). However, recent works have proposed that illness may not be related to the hard-*driving* Type A individual as much as to the *driven,* indicating that perception, sense of control, or some other coping factor may be more closely related to the maladaptive aspects of stress (Siegel, 1986). Also, some have characterized Type A personality qualities as a mediating variable rather than a characteristic from which stress originates (Holahan & Moos, 1985; Wheeler & Frank, 1988).

Lazarus (1966) discussed similar responses in reactions of fear, anger, depression, despair, hopelessness, and guilt. Operational definitions of stress fall on a continuum from simple nuisance to major threat or loss, with responses ranging from benign frustration to incapacitating grief. Such viewpoints of particular personality responses or characteristics generally dilute the precision of study and exclude the dimension of family interactions in examining stress from a family perspective. Personality characteristics are significant mediating variables in stress experiences, but must also be considered as important resources, as will be discussed later.

After decades of study, the same question—"What is stress?"—remains. However, recognizing the importance of the concept, and that it requires some tolerance of ambiguity as study evolves, researchers continue to move forward in explaining stress–coping phenomena, as will be described in subsequent chapters.

Coping

It is increasingly recognized that how people cope is the most significant mediating factor in the consequences of stress. The literature describes coping responses, strategies, styles, and resources (Dollahite, 1991), each with possible specific definitions. Throughout the evolution of the study of stress the identification of the concept of coping is noticeably absent.

While stress and coping have been recognized as interrelated, the definition of coping has eluded science even more than the definition of stress. Despite increasing interest in coping research, little is known about the nature or definition of coping, or how coping mediates the effects of stress. Selye's (1974) concept of adaptation resembles an idea of coping, as it appears to refer to accommodation to change and a desirable outcome of stress situations, but little attention has been given to coping processes, functions, or mediating factors.

Folkman and Lazarus (1980) asserted that the reason so little is known about coping is that "most coping research has been concerned with unusual populations . . . or with unusual or special events . . . that attention has not been given to the ways most people . . . cope with the ordinary stressful events of their day-to-day lives" (p. 219).

A new generation of scholars in the social sciences has promoted a current growing interest in the study of coping (see Antonovsky, 1979; Coelho, Hamberg, & Adams, 1974; Cohen, 1982; Folkman & Lazarus, 1980; Lazarus & Folkman, 1984; McCubbin, Larsen, & Olson, 1982; Menaghan, 1983; Panzarine, 1985). Though current stress research has progressed toward the recognition that coping is the significant factor in adaptation to stress, few studies have emphasized the coping component, and fewer still have given attention to coping with the ordinary stressors of daily life (Folkman & Lazarus, 1980; Lazarus & Folkman, 1984; Pearlin & Schooler, 1978).

Among the inquiries from a cognitive–phenomenological perspective of stressors and coping in well people is the work of Folkman (Folkman, 1979; Folkman & Lazarus, 1980). Although she considered adults aged 45–64, her theoretical foundation, rationale, and methodologies may offer a prototype for the analysis of children. In a population of 100 healthy, or "adequately functioning" adults, Folkman (1979) collected data related to daily stressors and coping responses through monthly interviews, self-report questionnaires between interviews, and the Ways of Coping checklist (Folkman & Lazarus, 1985) over a period of 1 year. Categorizing coping as problem- and emotion-focused, she analyzed the context of particular minor stressors, including persons involved, age, gender, mediators of coping, and consistency in coping patterns.

Folkman emphasized the need for data collection from particular described stressors in a naturalistic process rather than a trait orientation. The study offered an important landmark for scientific entry into the study of phenomenological approaches to stress and coping among people who seem to remain well. The Ways of Coping checklist also initiated attempts to measure coping from a process, rather than trait, approach.

The Coping Responses Scale was also developed following Lazarus's model (Moos, Cronkite, Billings, & Finney, 1984). Stability of the test has been studied in comparison with another test for use with ill adults (Roberts et al., 1987). As with Folkman's instrument, its use is limited to individual adults.

Klein (1983) explored relationships between family coping and family problem solving, noting:

> A family copes with a crisis by managing its affairs in whatever manner it can. . . . A family solves its problems by eliminating the difficulty. . . . There is the sense here in which crises, because of their severity, can only be assuaged, accepted, and handled on their own terms. Problems, on the other hand, are subject to control and eradication. (p. 88)

Following Klein's comparison, McCubbin and McCubbin (in press) present problem solving and coping together, with apparent conceptual synonymity, in their model of family resiliency.

In view of increasing interest in coping with stresses of daily life, or hassles, Klein's observation of the similarity between the concepts of "coping efficacy" and "problem-solving effectiveness" invokes an even broader arena of interdisciplinary study. We must consider variables closely related to coping, such as problem solving, in order to arrive at effective conceptual and clinical definitions of coping. A key issue is whether coping mediates the effects of stress, or is a response to those effects. Klein suggests that coping encompasses both concepts.

Boss (1988) argued that coping should be defined as cognitive, affective, and/or behavioral *management*. There is considerable current discussion regarding the concepts of management versus coping. Although the argument for use of the term management has some obvious merit, research has not yet clearly discriminated between the two terms. Thus, I will persist herein with the use of the term "coping," which is understood to encompass the concept of management. Most conceptual definitions of coping, following the cognitive–transactional framework, include management within the larger definition of coping itself. Indeed, Lazarus and Launier (1978) described coping as "efforts, both action-oriented and intrapsychic, to manage (i.e., master, tolerate, reduce, minimize) environmental and internal demands" (p. 311). Hereinafter, coping refers to all reported affective, behavioral, and interpersonal *responses* to stressors among the children and families of this study. Such a definition obviously includes the concept of management.

Coping is increasingly viewed as a process, rather than an event or trait. That is, coping is studied best by methods that explore the patterns of a person's continual appraisals, reappraisals, and actual responses in particular contexts, rather than isolated hypothetical responses of what he or she might do in a given situation. Thus, although particular coping styles have been examined (Holahan & Moos, 1985; Suls & Fletcher, 1985), the effectiveness of coping seems to depend more on repertoire than on style.

Appraisal

Growing interest in coping has paralleled inquiry into cognitive aspects of stress–coping phenomena. Individual cognitive appraisal, perception, or meaning of a stress event is increasingly viewed as a critical variable in stress responses (Lazarus & Folkman, 1984; McCubbin & Figley, 1983). Emphasis on the influence of individual and family appraisal opens the field beyond traditional conditioned-response or drive-forces theories toward more humanistic, holistic approaches to study. Boss (1987) emphasized that "the stressor event or situation does not act directly on the family system. Rather it is the perception of the event as mediated by internal and external contexts that determines whether the family will cope or fall into crisis" (p. 720).

Lazarus (1981) has presented a stress–coping paradigm that describes a transaction between the person and the environment, with perception or appraisal of the stressor as a key mediating factor. However, study of cognition related to stress responses in children is extremely limited (Brown, O'Keeffe, Sanders, & Baker, 1986; Walker, 1986). As will be discussed in the next chapter, McCubbin and associates (McCubbin, Sussman, & Patterson, 1983) have recognized the factor of appraisal as perception in family stress theory.

Coping Resources

There is increasing evidence that perception of stressors and the ways and effectiveness of coping are greatly influenced by the resources available. Coping resources, or stress buffers, are described here as mediating variables that reduce the effects of stressors or enhance coping. Resources may include personal characteristics, such as particular personality types, health, values and beliefs, sense of control, and skills. Material and environmental resources include money and access to services. Interpersonal resources include networks for social support. Kanner and associates (1981) have also recognized "uplifts," or positive daily events, that are viewed here as resources. Although such resources have been studied as individual variables, there is a need to learn about (1) the effects of individual perceptions of resources on stress outcomes, (2) children's perceptions of resources, and (3) the interrelated effects of resources on family variables.

In the past there has been less emphasis on coping than on measures of stress. However, recent interest in coping and related issues such as problem solving, appraisal, and resources has opened new avenues toward a better understanding of human adaptation.

Unfortunately, however, traditional lines of research have followed the long-accepted, limited perspectives and definitions of stress and coping. A brief review of such research follows.

NATURE OF THE PROBLEMS STUDIED

Traditional perceptions of stress and coping that largely followed the prevailing ideas of Selye (1974) have, until recently, resulted in fairly restricted lines of inquiry in research and practice. Traditional research is interpreted here in the following major categories: (1) correlational studies, associating stress with some type of pathology or other physiological response; (2) intervention studies, showing psychophysiological effects of various stress management, educational, or mediation techniques; (3) testing or identification of particular mediating variables or coping responses; and (4) gender issues, exploring the influence of differences between females and males in the study of stress–coping phenomena.

Correlation Studies

A large body of professional literature traces stress, usually defined by events scales, to physiological illness. Correlational studies have demonstrated relationships between stress and pathology or other physiological responses in nearly every system of the human organism. Indeed, there is some belief that all illness may be somehow related to stress (Davison & Neal, 1990; Monat & Lazarus, 1991). Though the focus of this book is on psychosocial stressors (generally as antecedent variables), the volume of work examining physiological stress, usually as the dependent variable, must be considered.

Life stress has been related to myocardial infarction and cerebral vascular accident (Friedman & Rosenman, 1974; Rahe, McKean, & Arthur, 1972), hypertension and other cardiovascular diseases (Brod, 1982), increased susceptibility to infection (Meyer & Haggerty, 1962), increased complications of pregnancy (Nuckolls, Cassel, & Kaplan, 1972), and increased use of medical services in general among families (Roghmann & Haggerty, 1972). Other physical disorders associated with stress include bronchial asthma, gastric ulcers, hyperthyroidism, diabetes (Price, 1985), and decreased immune response, and cancer (Levy, 1982).

Stress-associated mental disorders include depression and drug abuse. Stress has also been associated with suicide (Bieliauskas, 1982). Decreased employee health and productivity have been attributed to stress (Cooper, 1983; Seamonds, 1982), and positive correlations have even been demonstrated between life stresses and criminal behavior (Levinson & Ramsey, 1979; Masuda, Culter, Hein, & Holmes, 1978).

Though studies are fewer, the stress–illness relationship has also been demonstrated among children (Johnson, 1986). The majority of studies correlating stress and illness have relied on life-change events scales as measurements of stress. Such studies, which focus on the maladaptive effects of isolated or multiple traumatic events, by their nature and design overlook individual appraisal or perception and individual or family adaptive or coping phenomena. Call (1983) claimed that the traditional positive relationship between life events and illness is typically of low clinical significance, suggesting the need for study of mediating variables.

There have been few examinations of those people who do not demonstrate maladaptive responses to stress, the more ordinary common stressors of daily life, or the individual or family appraisal of stressors. Haggerty (1980) pointed out that a majority of families do not respond to stress by increased illness and identified a need for analysis of "forces that lead to positive health, rather than only those that lead to illness" (p. 395), and investigation of factors that prevent the maladaptive results of stress, or that may protect the individual from the illness-producing results of stressful life events. In 1981, Miller asserted that future studies in stress and coping must "assess the full range of psychological components that account for adjusted persons" and study the effects of stress "on a range of different types of people" (p. 320) and on individual differences. As mentioned, even Selye (1983) acknowledged a "good stress" (eustress), which led not to illness but rather to "fulfillment" (p. 18).

In short, correlations between stress and illness or maladaptation, though numerous and valid, have been restricted to a few variables of study, restricted definitions of stress, and limited populations. There is a need for more inclusive models of study.

Intervention Studies

A second type of stress–coping literature concentrates on behavioral, educational, or cognitive stress-intervention techniques for various psychophysiological parameters of stress or coping. Numerous programs incorporating one or more types of stress-management technique—such as time management, biofeedback, guided imagery, meditation, various methods of relaxation, assertive communication, thought stopping, or other behavioral training, environmental condition, or cognitive or social education component—have been proposed to reduce the maladaptive effects of stress (see Curtis & Detert, 1981; Jencks, 1979; McKay, Davis, & Fanning, 1981; Woolfolk & Lehrer, 1984; Woolfolk, Lehrer, McCann, & Roonery, 1982). Monat and Lazarus (1991) categorized such programs according to their purpose to (1) alter environment and/or lifestyle, (2) alter personality characteristics and/or perception, or (3) alter biological responses to stress.

Empirical evidence regarding the effectiveness of such programs is sparse. Actually, most literature on stress management concentrates on the "how to" of untested programs, rather than reporting whether or not they work. One issue is the limited measures of dependent variables as outcomes of stress-management interventions. Rather than examining the effect on coping or adaptation, the research among such programs, usually following Selye's theory, uses indirect measurements, such as blood pressure, muscle tension, heart rate, or self-reported feelings of well-being. Long-term effects of such stress-management interventions on daily life or even any immediate value in subsequent acute real-life stressor situations remain unknown. Further, there is a need for scientific determination of the most effective focus for intervention. That is, we must know when interventions are most effectively directed at modifying stressors, changing perceptions, or teaching coping or management skills.

Monat and Lazarus (1991) asserted that while such interventions may not cause harm, it has not been shown to what extent, or even whether or not, stress management techniques actually work. Further, they cautioned that professional promotion of unvalidated cures by a stress management "industry," consisting of consultants and self-help presentations, may trivialize or commercialize the distress of life.

While some stress-management programs have been proposed for children (Englehardt, 1986; Hendricks & Wills, 1975; LaMontagne et al., 1985), their validity in terms of the assessment of coping or the long-term effects on coping remains open for study. Most interventions for children have been developed from adult models, based on assumptions about adult subjects without validation from the direct perspective of the child. Still to be examined are the effectiveness of stress-management techniques over time, programs that promote a repertoire of coping possibilities, and the need for a variety of stress-management interventions that accommodate individual differences. Furthermore, most stress-intervention techniques are directed at particular individual responses, and do not accommodate the realities of daily life, interactions within families, or responses within the family as a unit.

Studies of Coping Resources or Mediating Variables

The third major type of investigation has been the testing or identification of particular mediating variables, or coping resources, associated with stress. Such mediating variables have been called "stress buffers." These factors are generally conceptualized as personal or situational characteristics that mediate stressor effects or assist in coping efforts (Sorensen, 1991; Wheeler & Frank, 1988).

Two frequently studied stress buffers that most commonly mediate in stress–coping situations related to illness are (1) social support (see Cassel, 1976; Cobb, 1976; Cohen & Wills, 1985; Haggerty, 1980; Moos, 1974; Norbeck, 1981; Schilling, Gilchrist, & Schinke, 1984;

Thoits, 1986) and (2) individual sense of control (Langer, 1975), including locus of control (see Gilbert, 1976; Kilmann, Laval, & Wanlass, 1978; Parkes, 1984; Rothbaum, Wolfer, & Visintainer, 1979; Rotter, 1966). Wheeler and Frank (1988) noted that the greatest controversy over social support and control concerned the overwhelming use of life events as the measure of stress.

Rejecting life events in favor of daily hassles as measures of stress, other researchers advanced the concept of "uplifts," defined as "positive or satisfying experiences" that are a counterpart of hassles (DeLongis et al., 1982; Kanner et al., 1981). The conceptual relationship between buffers and uplifts has not been explored.

Kobasa and associates (Kobasa, 1979; 1982; Kobasa, Maddi, & Courington, 1981; Kobasa, Maddi, & Kahn, 1982) proposed a particular personality characteristic termed "hardiness" as a stress–coping mediator. They identified the characteristics of hardiness as personal control, commitment, and challenge. However, such data have largely been drawn from populations of middle-aged, middle-class males. Although there have been some limited attempts to establish the validity of the hardiness construct in females (McCranie, Lambert, & Lambert, 1987), data among children or families are sparse. Limited use of the original concept of hardiness with families has resulted in some revision (Failla & Jones, 1991; McCubbin, McCubbin, & Thompson, 1986).

Pollock (1986) adapted Kobasa's definition of hardiness to a more health-specific orientation, expanding the concept to include elements of physiological and psychological adaptation. Pollock (1989) further recognized the important role of personal appraisal in the quality of hardiness. Questions remain about the definition and validity of the construct (Lee, 1983; Wagnild & Young, 1991).

The variable of "resilience" (Garmezy, 1991; Leonard, 1991; Patterson, 1991; Sinnema, 1991), studied to a limited extent among children and families, resembles the concept of hardiness. Resilience, social competence, and coping have been studied as variables related to hardiness in children's abilities to endure life stress.

Many other physiological, behavioral, psychosocial, and environmental factors have been identified as stress–coping mediating factors. Physiological factors include immune-system characteristics (Levy, 1982). Buffering behavioral practices related to stress include health and lifestyle practices (Wiebe & McCallum, 1986), such as daily routines, nutrition, and physical fitness (Roth & Holmes, 1985).

Psychosocial buffers include individual characteristics, such as vulnerability (Gottschalk, 1983; Murphy & Moriarty, 1976), meaningfulness, congruency, self-complexity and self-esteem (Linville, 1987; Witmer, Rich, Barcikowski, & Mague, 1983), and temperament (Garmezy & Rutter, 1983). Other factors include mental load, fatigue, arousal, individual differences, and sense of ambiguity (Friedman, 1982; Holt, 1982; Steinmetz, Kaplan, & Miller, 1982). The positive characteristics of optimism (Scheier, Weintraub, & Carver, 1986) and humor (Martin & Lefcourt, 1983) have been recognized and popularized (Cousins, 1976; Siegel, 1986).

Buffers such as specific environmental conditions (Holt, 1982), person–environment fit (Caplan, Naidu, & Tripathi, 1984; Matteson & Ivancevich, 1982), and particular occupations have also been examined.

Most of these stress buffers have scarcely been studied in children or family units, with the exception of some work exploring family strengths (McCubbin, 1989). Most works have examined urban, Western, middle-aged, middle-class adults. Inquiries among children have generally focused on particular risk situations or traumatic life events, such as illness, hospitalization, loss as in death or divorce, or stress-producing conditions such as having an ill sibling, or being classified as gifted. Among the few exceptions that have explored, to a limited extent, some mediating factors in healthy children are those examining developmental transitions, such as adolescence (Mechanic, 1983; Price, 1985), and the work on resilience, temperament, social competence, and vulnerability.

Wheeler and Frank (1988) outlined several problematic issues in the traditional study of stress buffers. They observed that (1) buffer studies generally consider only single or limited groups of variables, precluding important comparisons, (2) the over-used measure of life events for stress ignores other important components of the stress construct, particularly individual perception, (3) the measure of health has been inadequately defined based on limited lists of symptoms, and (4) analytical procedures have failed to differentiate between main and interaction effects, with occasionally misleading results. These issues are compounded in the study of children and families.

Although buffers may complicate research designs and clutter potential theoretical models, they may indeed comprise the most important variables for valid results. Buffers seem to be strongly related to process, appraisal, and individual or family differences, and very influential in outcomes. Positive buffers, such as resilience, hardiness, and family strengths need to be included in family stress-coping equations. Certainly, they must be considered as study progresses toward intervention development. However, it remains to be discovered whether these resources are best conceptualized as aspects of stress experiences, characteristics of individuals or families, or integral aspects of coping responses.

Gender Issues

Traditional research has not highlighted gender issues in stress–coping phenomena. As in the case with stress-management techniques, gender factors have seemed to command more attention in lay literature than in empirical studies (Witkin-Lanoil, 1984, 1986). Until recently, as in other health and psychosocial research, mainstream stress–coping studies of individuals have been mainly conducted with middle-aged, middle-class white males. Examples include the early evolution of such constructs as Type A behavior and hardiness. Men appear to be overrepresented in the study of stressors, while women have been overrepresented in research on social networks (Belle, 1991). Belle further found that although some research has focused on single-sex groups, such as women in reproductive and family roles, or men in occupational roles, few analyses have concentrated on gender differences in particular.

Bolger, DeLongis, Kessler, and Wethington (1989) studied stress in multiple roles among husbands and wives. They found that husbands were more likely than wives to bring stress from home into the workplace, and that wives were more likely than husbands to accommodate and modify home demands to compensate for the work-related stresses of spouses.

Ironically, the most attention given to gender differences in stress and coping is found in studies of children and adolescents. Those works will be reviewed in later chapters.

More examination of gender-related factors is found in recent investigations of stress-moderating variables. There is some evidence that a stronger stress–illness relationship exists for women, perhaps because women seem to somatize more than men (Matheny & Cupp, 1983). Folkman and Lazarus (1980) noted that women reported more stressful daily events related to health and family, while men reported more stressful work-related episodes. However, no significant gender differences were distinguished in coping responses. Men used more problem-focused coping than women, but only at work. No differences in the use of emotion-focused coping were evident.

Researchers who developed hassles scales discovered interesting gender-related associations. More powerful associations between hassles and social–emotional adjustment were found among women and, ironically, women exhibited a positive correlation between uplifts (positive daily life events) and undesirable outcomes (Kanner et al., 1981). Thus it appears that women both experience more daily negative stressors and are better able to perceive positive influences than men.

The stress mediator of social support seems to have attracted the most examination of gender implications. Belle (1987, 1991) concluded from her review of gender issues in social moderators of stress that women mobilize and rely on social support more during stress, and that women are *providers* of more frequent and effective social support than men, perhaps reciprocally becoming more vulnerable to stress. Others have validated that women's propensity to more intimate human relationships may increase a sensitivity to the stressors of others. Such sensitivity can be reflected as a personal vulnerability to stress and a risk to a woman's own health (Kessler & McLeod, 1984; Wethington, McLeod, & Kessler, 1987).

There remains much to be learned about gender implications in stress-coping phenomena among adults. Gender issues in children and families will be discussed later.

IMPLICATIONS FOR RESEARCH OF CHILDREN AND FAMILIES

The "individual" or "organism" to which most definitions refer is frequently applied to aggregates or systems, such as the family unit, though such application invokes questions of theoretical and empirical validity. The concepts of stress events or daily hassles as measures of stress become even more complex and interactional if considered from the viewpoint of individuals in a family. It also becomes even more difficult to measure responses from the complex informant of a family as a single unit. The critical variables of perception, appraisal, cognition, and coping become unwieldy, as the "family response," representing either the sum of its members or some compound equation, is sought. However, such variables need to be studied from the perspective of the family.

Furthermore, antecedents and outcomes become more complex as one studies individual factors, family factors, and other social factors as they interrelate with individual stress and family stress. For example, the stress of an individual family member may influence the health or outcome of the family unit, or problems within the family may influence individual functioning.

Most of the research cited in this chapter has simply ignored the powerful variable of family. In traditional research, though correlation studies have included some family groups, studies of intervention techniques or of mediating variables have most often been applied to individuals, or representative members of families.

On the other hand, family researchers cannot measure factors of the family unit if they avoid considering existing knowledge of stress–coping phenomena in individuals, or refuse to include viewpoints of particular individuals in the family unit. For example, Burr, Burr, and Holman (in press) justified the exclusion of any consideration of Lazarus's models of stress–coping by stating that "his approach is an individualistic psychologic approach that deals with individual's stress" (p. 58). They then appeared to reinvent the concepts of process, subjective appraisal, and coping strategies from a "family" perspective, as if they were independent of consideration of the individuals that comprise families.

Another common example appears in Lavee and Olson's (1991) study, where they assert that "only the husbands' and wives' data were used, since adding a third . . . person's data, in only a portion of the sample, would have greatly increased the complexity of the study" (p. 789). I submit that such complexity is the essential reality of research about families. There is a need for multidisciplinary collaboration and dissolution of ostensible boundaries between theoretical territories. Integrated theories that can account for all variables must be developed.

SUMMARY AND CONCLUSIONS

The perspective or viewpoint of a study must be recognized in such complex issues of stress–coping phenomena, and among complex groups of subjects, such as children and families. Units of analysis, both as antecedent and consequential variables need to be acknowledged and identified. In addition, the analytical matrix that includes definition of terms, units of observation, and epistemological assumptions ought to be outlined.

Traditional definitions and interpretations of stress were explored, including the related terms "life events" and "hassles," and other measures that lay the historical foundation for current study. More recent interpretations of coping, appraisal, and resources were presented.

Traditional research, using the outlined definitions, was divided into the three major categories of correlational studies, intervention studies, and the testing of mediating variables, with an additional examination of gender issues.

Regarding stress and coping, traditional literature generally reveals the following: (1) the emphasis of study has been among populations of individuals at risk for particular sources of stress, focusing on stressors rather than on coping responses; (2) stress has been cast largely as major life-change events, although the phenomena of daily life seem to affect health and illness more; (3) methods have been limited to quantitative approaches that often ignore subjective reports or issues such as individual or gender differences as compounding variables; and (4) most studies have fallen short of examining the realities of the individual within a family context or considering the dynamics of the family as a unit.

A brief preview of the implications for research on children and families revealed that while traditional efforts have provided some attention to stress–coping variables, there remain many areas for examination, particularly from the phenomenological viewpoint of children in families.

The Family Perspective:
Theoretical
and Methodological Notes

An understanding of individual perception and behavior is grounded in a knowledge of the family context from which the individual emerges. First, family phenomena offer important antecedent and dependent variables in studies of individual stress and coping. Second, there is significant current discussion, referring to the family as a unit of study, about "family perceptions" and "family responses" (Boss, 1988; Feetham, 1984; Gilliss, 1983; Draper & Marcos, 1990; Litman, 1974; Uphold & Strickland, 1989). For both these reasons, the study of stress–coping phenomena among children is invalid without consideration of the family unit.

Explorations of stress and coping in children have traditionally been conducted within the context of school or therapy. Few studies have examined such phenomena in the natural setting of the home from the multilateral viewpoint of the family. Thus, this chapter will explore largely the "family perspective on families," described in the previous chapter. Issues related more specifically to children will be considered in the next chapter.

GENERAL THEORETICAL FOUNDATIONS

Theoretical foundations that establish a body of knowledge in family study, contributing to several disciplines, have emerged and flourished in recent decades (Beutler, Burr, Bahr, & Herrin, 1989; Broderick, 1971; Burr, Hill, Nye, & Reiss, 1979). Indeed, family study has recently indulged in considerable "theorizing about theory," that is, self-analysis of the process of family theory building and research.

Examples include the works of Sprey (1988), Lavee and Dollahite (1991), Beutler and colleagues (1989), and Burr, Herrin, Day, Beutler, and Leigh (1988). Theory is also being developed in clinical practices such as nursing (Clements & Roberts, 1983; Gilliss, Highley, Roberts, & Martinson, 1989; Whall, 1980, 1981; Whall & Fawcett, 1991). Such reflection, including the consideration of metatheory, indicates active, productive, though perhaps conflicted, scientific activity (Klein & Jurich, in press). Such active intellectual inquiry provokes a need for similarly active multidisciplinary approaches to the study of the family.

The family has been described as a system of interacting personalities bound by biology, rules, and ritual (Boss, 1988); an entity greater than, or different from, the sum of its parts (Gilliss, 1983; White, 1984); and unique in ethics, processes, and dynamics among all other aspects of human experience (Beutler et al., 1989).

Study of the family as a unit and of family phenomena has expanded across the social sciences, initially guided by general theories developed in disciplines other than what may be currently called family sciences (Beutler et al., 1989). Such theories, originating largely in sociology, usually viewed family phenomena as dependent variables. Three decades ago, Hill and Hansen (1960) identified five frameworks for family study: interactional, structural–functional, situational, institutional, and developmental. During the 1970s, other approaches, such as balance, game, and exchange theories, emerged. Burr and associates (1979) integrated some middle-range theories with the more developed family theories of social exchange, symbolic interaction, general systems, conflict, and phenomenology. In 1980, Holman and Burr described and assigned status ratings to the family theories mentioned above, in addition to theories of psychoanalysis, field, learning, behaviorism, and ecosystems.

Other theories associated with the study of the family include role, attachment, conflict, crisis, and various communication theories (Clements & Roberts, 1983). There is an emerging interest in family study among nurses, and the works of several scholars identify and develop concepts from existing theories in nursing that are related to the family (Clements & Roberts, 1983; Whall & Fawcett, 1991).

Though it is not the purpose of this work to comprehensively review or evaluate theoretical perspectives in family study, the potential relevance of a few major theories is explored. Even if particular theories do not drive research, it is important to recognize and acknowledge significant philosophical and theoretical influences. Kaplan (1964) asserted that "no human perception is immaculate" (pp. 131–132), and that "no observation can be undertaken in all innocence.

We always know something already, and this knowledge is intimately involved in what we come to know next, whether by [purposeful] observation or in any other way."

Some current frameworks that are relevant to family research and practice and to stress–coping phenomena include interactionist, developmental, systems, and social exchange theories. These are explored and compared more extensively by Mercer (1989). These theories are also useful in the study of children.

Symbolic Interactionism

The interactionist perspective is based on assumptions of the meanings of symbols and on the introspective and reflexive abilities of human beings. It allows for processes, rather than products of family social interactions, and assumes that behavior is influenced by symbolic meaning, rather than instincts or drives. Meanings and values are derived partially through social interactions (Burr, Leigh, Day, & Constantine, 1979; Gallant & Kleinman, 1983; Maurin, 1983). The emergence of "a universe of shared meanings" (Maurin, 1983, p. 99) is a distinctive characteristic and a requirement for sustained interaction, as well as a part of the culture of a family. Dissonance and/or synchrony in shared meanings influence the quality of the human experience (O'Neill, & Sorensen, 1991). Another important assumption in the symbolic interactionist perspective is the human process of continual selective interpretation, deliberation, and action, in contrast to stimulus–response models (Knafl & Grace, 1978).

The interactionist philosophy can be broadly applied to qualitatively explain a large range of family phenomena. The approach lends itself well to the helping professions for description and comparison of phenomena and has been used in a variety of studies of family issues (Corbin & Strauss, 1985; Roberts, 1983; Ventura & Stevenson, 1986). Its qualitative viewpoint, which focuses on dynamic relationships among family members (Klein, 1983) and values the subjective meanings of each member of the family, is conducive to the inclusion of children as valuable informants in family study.

Elements of symbolic interactionism are evident in several family theories. For example, the "C factor" of family perception, defined loosely as "family-specific meaning," seems in Hill's (1958) and McCubbin's (McCubbin & Patterson, 1983) ABCX models for family stress/crisis to be subtly influenced by symbolic interactionist philosophy.

In my own study, concepts from symbolic interactionism inspired the search for symbolic meaning from the subjective viewpoint of children and parents and from children's expressions in art. Though I did not set out with a symbolic interactionist orientation, this philosophy certainly influenced some of my assumptions about symbolic meaning in children. Subtle symbolic interactionist influences are evident in the design of the study, as well as in the approach to data analysis, as the child's perspective on meaning was interpreted from symbols offered by children themselves, and as dissonance or synchrony were sought in analysis of parent, child, and sometimes sibling diary reports.

Developmental Theory

Mercer (1989) argued that though the developmental approach draws from other foundations, such as symbolic interactionist, systems, structural–functional, psychoanalytic, and cognitive theories, the perspective offers unique philosophical and methodological characteristics. Families are comprised of individuals whose separate development influences the organization, adaptation, and development of the family system. Classic developmental theorists who have influenced family study include Erikson, Freud, and Piaget. Modern developmentalists include Duvall (1957), Havighurst (1972), Rodgers (1964), Werner (1948), Hill (1966), and Aldous (1990). The general philosophy of the developmental framework describes a general (continuous or discontinuous) movement of family members, and thus the family unit, to higher levels of functioning, with reversion to lower levels during transitions or traumas of disequilibrium. The notion of the life cycle of a family, with predictable stages and developmental tasks, provides fairly discrete time periods and/or units for study. However, the validity of some assumptions related to those units may be questionable. For example, an adolescent single-parent family may offer very different developmental variables than the two-parent family described by traditional developmental theory.

Since developmental theory assumes particular processes over time, it is best accommodated and tested by longitudinal designs. While the theory may include developmental implications for the entire family unit, its application seems most frequently applied to specific family age-groups or transitions, such as early parenthood or child rearing. Problems seem to emerge in measurement of individual and family group variables, where developmental asynchrony can confound outcomes. Researchers then often revert to a limited, single-informant view of the family, usually a parental perception, though this approach is not confined to developmental research.

There also appear to be limitations in studying the many dimensions of lateral traumatic phenomena, such as divorce, chronic illness of a family member, daily individual struggles, or events in a nontraditional family structure. These problems may be due to inadequate tools to describe, measure, or predict development in such situations.

However, developmental theory, by definition, suggests that variables in the study of stress and coping in children include a significant age or developmental dependence. Indeed, any important study of phenomena in the lives of school-age children would be expected to include a developmental viewpoint to some degree. Developmental theory provides a context that may shape children's perceptions of stressors as well as influence coping styles or repertoires, and suggests the distribution of such characteristics across different ages. It also allows for the effects of stress–coping events and patterns of early childhood on adult functioning.

With few exceptions (Altshuler & Ruble, 1989; Stern, 1990), though child researchers have implied a developmental approach, development has not been directly addressed as a variable in stress–coping research among children. Unfortunately, the ostensible developmental approach to research with children seldom goes beyond attention to age.

Developmental theory in research about children may seem mature, as various age-group tasks and levels of functioning, along with associated concepts and propositions, have been well identified and tested. However, the fairly new idea of a unique culture of childhood offers challenges in renewed concept development and empirical application. Certainly, attention to the age and developmental expectations of school-age children contributed to assumptions about data collection measures in my study.

General Systems Theory

General systems theory has applications in many scientific disciplines. Bertalanffy's (1950, 1968) classic works describe open systems that exchange matter and energy with the environment, moving dynamically toward greater order, satisfaction, or complexity of the system. The isolated closed system then moves toward increased disorder, disintegration, and entropy. An open system can maintain a state of homeostasis by the circular processes of feedback. Fawcett (1975) called the family a loving open system, and Rogers (1983) described the family as "an irreducible energy field, different from its parts [members] and manifesting characteristics that cannot be predicted from knowledge of (individual) members" (p. 226). Systems theory promotes a process, rather than outcome, orientation, depicting the family as it relates and interacts with other systems thus allowing a more holistic approach.

Systems theory is conducive to model building, elicits complex data-analytic methods, and sometimes may appear to distance the investigator from the lived realities of families, toward more academic, esoteric explanations of family phenomena. However, this is not to say that systems theory is not applicable in accommodating the complex family interactions evident in stress–coping phenomena, particularly when studying the child's viewpoint. Indeed, systems theory offers conceptual mechanisms for viewing both individual (child and/or adult) and family variables within a unified context. While systems theory did not contribute directly to my research, the framework certainly became salient after data were analyzed.

Social Exchange Theory

The classic work of Homans (1958), drawing from economic theories, proposed that family interactions might be viewed as an exchange of material and nonmaterial goods. General principles of social exchange theory are that individual rewards within a group are reciprocal, that greater cohesiveness in the group leads to greater value in the exchange among members of the group, that individuals within the group make choices that result in "greatest rewards at the least cost" (Mercer, 1989, p. 28), and that individual satisfaction and family equilibrium are achieved if there is reciprocity whereby goods match the value in costs.

Social exchange theory has been used to study family decision making, mate selection, divorce, power, social policy, and family violence. The implied elements of individual appraisal, negotiation, and change may have merit for the study of children's perceptions of family responses to stress and may help to explain interdependence among family members.

However, there may be a risk in not including the aspects of human relationships that reflect exchanges outside the concept of reciprocity. Therefore, although a social exchange orientation provides some direction, it cannot provide the entire foundation for the study of stress and coping in children and families and offered little to my own study, except as a possible framework for explaining some exchanges and comparisons among parent–child dyads.

There is some evidence that scholars are now attempting to tie family stress–coping theory to other family theories, like those described above. Other theories related to family functioning may also contribute to knowledge of family responses to stressful episodes. For example, the Circumflex Model (Lavee & Olson, 1991; Olson, 1985; Olson, Sprenkle, & Russell, 1979) focuses on dimensions of family cohesion and family adaptability. The model has been used to identify particular family types. Such theoretical integrations are beginning to influence empirical studies.

Despite admirable efforts in theory development, theoretical adequacy and conceptual clarity have been of major concern in family research (Gilliss, 1983; Gochman, 1985; Haley, 1972; Litman & Venters, 1979; Riskin & Faunce, 1972). While the literature offers an outpouring of family studies, often "the concept of family is not defined within the framework of the research, nor is the family the basic unit of analysis in the research" (Feetham, 1984, p. 6). Further, there is no consensus on the most appropriate model for study (Gochman, 1985). Some researchers caution that most theories continue to overlook the uniqueness of phenomena related to "the family realm" (Beutler et al., 1989; Burr et al., 1988).

THEORETICAL FOUNDATIONS IN STRESS–COPING PHENOMENA

Friedman (1992) asserted that no single theory fully describes family phenomena, and recognized a need for an eclectic approach, particularly in clinical practice. In 1973, Burr attempted to synthesize the family stress propositions and theories developed to that time. Burr recognized several important mediating variables and stressor influences, such as familism in extended families, marital adjustment, activity of wives outside the home, and power structures of spouses. However, the influences of children as informants, child sibling relationships, or even child-related variables, beyond their effect on the adults of the family, were largely absent. Such concepts need to be defined, and their role as variables in family stress theory need to be outlined.

Recently, several other scholars have proposed the integration of various theories related to family stress and coping. For example, Burr and colleagues (in press) proposed the integration of stress–coping theory with systems theory; Dollahite (1991) has linked family stress theory with theories in family resource management; and Koop and Keating (1990) suggested the integration of the ABCX model with the cognitive–transactional model. Even in these more recent theory connections, the child is apparently absent, except as an antecedent stressor variable (such as the chronically ill child). There is a specific need to include minor children as valued informants, and a general need for further development and empirical testing of concepts and propositions.

Acknowledging the influence of the frameworks already described herein, along with the daunting contribution of Hans Selye (1956, 1974), two theories contributed the most to the design and analysis of my study. The works of Hill (1949), revised and refined by McCubbin and colleagues (1980), and the efforts of Lazarus (1966) provided the foundation for an integrated theoretical approach.

ABCX Theory

Foundations for current theoretical models specific to stress–coping phenomena in families began with Burgess (1926), Angell (1936), Koos (1946), and Hill (1949). Hill's (1958) classic ABCX theory for family stress or crisis has served as the predominant model in family stress research. Essentially, interacting variables are described as A (the stressor event and attending hardships), B (the family's resources), and C (the family's definition, perception, or meaning of the event), all of which interact to produce and contribute to X (the crisis).

Hill further described a course of family adjustment that includes (1) an initial period of disorganization, (2) a state of recovery, and (3) achievement of a new level of organization (Hill, 1949; McCubbin et al., 1980). The framework has been modified as research has evolved (Burr, 1973; McCubbin & McCubbin, 1987, in press; McCubbin & Patterson, 1983).

McCubbin and associates (McCubbin & Patterson, 1983) revised Hill's ABCX model to better reflect the realities of family stress. They noted that the original model only detailed precrisis variables influencing family capabilities for resistance or adaptation to stressor events. The revised double ABCX model considers family resiliency, recovery efforts over time, additional stressors or changes that pile up and influence coping abilities, family resources, and outcomes.

Double ABCX theory (McCubbin & Patterson, 1983) adds several factors. The aA factor represents strains, hardships, and "pileups" of stressors that affect a family, in addition to the primary stress event.

Such strains could originate from the initial stressor and its hardships, normative family transitions, previous and concurrent family problems or strains, consequences of family coping efforts, or from conditions of ambiguity or uncertainty. Such demands emerge from within individual family members, from within the family system, and/or from the community environment.

Some researchers have attempted to interpret and use Hill's and McCubbin's variable A in various family stressor categories, such as normative, volitional, nonvolitional, chronic, or acute (Boss, 1988). However, such assessment of family stressors becomes difficult without considering the personal appraisal of the family members (the C factor), or other variables such as duration, severity, or ambiguity.

Family resources (bB factors) are viewed as capabilities to resist disruption and promote adaptation to a stressor event. Such resources may include the intrinsic characteristics of the family, such as nurturance, role structure understanding and flexibility, and shared values. Environmental resources include such factors as economic capability, social support, and religious affiliation.

The cC factors represent the family's subjective definition and meaning of stressor events. From a clinical viewpoint, the C variable of family perception of the stressor event appears to be the most significant and powerful factor. However, family perception and appraisal, along with coping, remain the least investigated (Boss, 1987). Although McCubbin and associates (1980) viewed perception as a central variable, they expressed the difficulty of identifying the *source* of perception, asking:

> If there is a family "collective" perception, is parental perception the most important; under what conditions do children's perceptions become critical; and do discrepancies in perception among members need to be examined or considered, and when? (p. 862)

These questions remain largely unanswered.

The notion of the convergence of individual perceptions of different family members is a complex issue that merits more study. Reiss (1981) has attempted to use the concept of "shared construing," that is, the characteristics of a family, not the sum of its parts, that represent specific shared orientations, explanations, and comprehension relating to the internal and external environments that influence the body of the family. Lavee and Olson (1991) have also explored perceptions and responses of the family unit according to "family type."

According to McCubbin and Patterson (1983), factor xX represents family crisis as only one phase in the progression of family adjustment, introducing the concept of postcrisis adjustment and adaptation.

McCubbin and McCubbin (1987) later revised the model to depict phases of adjustment and adaptation and to include additional factors of family vulnerability, family typology, adaptive coping and family regenerativity. With these changes, adaptation represents both process and outcomes.

The McCubbins have recently further refined their model, in their resiliency model of family stress, adjustment, and adaptation to include several phases that represent the family's adjustment and adaptation processes over time. They now recognize additional factors, beyond those represented by A, B, C, and X, including vulnerability, family types and patterns, and problem solving and coping (McCubbin & McCubbin, in press).

The double ABCX model has become the leading framework for examining family responses to major life events, crisis, and family trauma. However, though the model has met significant heuristic needs, it does not provide for complete understanding of family processes under stress, nor of the "multiple interdependent levels of the social system" (Walker, 1985, p. 827). Koop and Keating (1990) argued that the model appeared to suggest that a family must experience crisis in order to achieve adaptation; that several precrisis variables, such as pileup, coping, and resources should also be included in the postcrisis phase. Their most significant criticisms seem to be the model's inability to adequately accommodate processes over time and its increasing complexity.

Boss (1987) further noted the need to build on past theory but to move away from positivistic influences toward qualitative analyses. Burr and colleagues (in press) also criticized the theory for its encumbering positivistic roots. They proposed a revision that would move away from the propensity to encourage the development of causal laws toward a process orientation. However, they fell short of proposing a phenomenological perspective since they embraced systems theory.

To study the daily life stress of children in families, there is still a need for (1) consideration and integration of the perceptions of all family members, (2) recognition of the clinical significance of daily hassles (beyond their presence in pileup), and (3) more specific and comprehensive definitions of coping factors, as McCubbin and Patterson's (1983) descriptions were originally limited largely to the coping responses of avoidance, elimination, and assimilation. Later, coping definitions seemed to become more unwieldy, as other elements— problem solving, strategies, styles, behaviors, and procurement and use of resources to maintain, manage, or resolve stressor situations—were included (Koop & Keating, 1990; McCubbin & McCubbin, 1987). There is also a need to conceptualize family stress and coping as they influence stress and coping in the individual child.

A difficulty in using a positivistic model such as ABCX to outline family stress–coping phenomena is the apparent necessity of the model's increasing complexity. Thus, Koop and Keating argued for the integration of a more parsimonious approach offered by Lazarus's cognitive–transactional paradigm.

Cognitive-Transactional Theory

The cognitive–phenomenological paradigm (Lazarus, 1981; Lazarus & Folkman, 1984; Monat & Lazarus, 1991) defines stress as a particular relationship between the person or family system and the environment that is appraised as taxing or exceeding resources and endangering well-being.

Individual perception, or cognitive appraisal, is a key factor in the cognitive–transactional framework. Lazarus (1982) proposed that cognitive processes "generate, influence, and shape" (p. 1024) human response and that cognitive activity is a necessary precondition to emotional response (Lazarus, 1984a). Cognitive appraisal, although not implying "deliberate reflection, rationality, or awareness" (Lazarus, 1982, p. 1022), "is an evaluative process that determines why and to what extent a particular transaction or series of transactions between the person and environment is stressful" (Lazarus & Folkman, 1984, p. 19). An event is evaluated according to "what is at stake" (primary appraisal) and what coping resources and options are available (secondary appraisal) (Folkman & Lazarus, 1980, p. 223).

Elements of cognitive appraisal and adaptation are also found in cognitive adaptation theory (Behr, Murphy, & Summers, 1992; Taylor, 1983; Taylor & Brown, 1988), which proposes that some individuals respond to threatening events through a process of cognitive adjustment that includes a reframing or even an illusionary resolution of life stress. Illusions do not represent a denial of facts, but a way of appraising situations in a positive, acceptable view. Cognitive themes in such a process include a search for the meaning of the stressor event, attempts to achieve mastery or control, and attempts to enhance personal self-esteem.

Coping is proposed as the "process through which the individual manages the demands of the person–environment relationship that are appraised as stressful and the emotions they generate" (Lazarus & Folkman, 1984, p. 19). Three types of coping efforts have been identified: (1) problem focused, or the "management or alteration of the person–environment relationship that is the source of stress," (2) emotion focused, or the regulation of stressful emotions, and (3) a combination of problem focused and emotion focused (Folkman & Lazarus, 1980, p. 223). Identification and description of coping strategies are prerequisite to the needed study of the effectiveness of particular coping responses and patterns, or the significance of particular coping repertoires.

Stress, appraisal, and coping are elements of dynamic interactive processes, termed "transactions" because both the person and the environment may mutually or reciprocally influence each other. Such a view proposes a "de-emphasis of predominantly structure or trait orientation toward the events intervening between the person and the environment, and an increasing emphasis on a process orientation centering on the person's continuing relationship with the environment" (Lazarus, 1981, p. 180).

This transactional view focuses on the process of a continuous flow of events over time as the person, with responses of appraisal and coping, and environment continually interchange with each other. Obviously, what may be appraised as stressful by one person may not be perceived as such by another. What is debilitating to one may be exhilarating to another. Though stress–coping processes and outcomes have been described as adaptive or maladaptive, such concepts are obviously dependent upon individual interpretation, effects, and value systems, as well as environmental factors.

Lazarus and Folkman (1984) observed that "the ways people actually cope also depend heavily on the resources that are available to them and the constraints that inhibit use of these resources in the context of the specific encounter" (p. 158). Coping resources are viewed as mediating variables interacting with the person and the environment, influencing the stress–coping process. Lazarus and Folkman (1984) listed the following examples of individual coping resources: health and energy, positive beliefs, problem-solving skills, social skills, social support, and material resources.

Methodological Tenets

Lazarus suggested four major methodological tenets for the study of stress and coping: (1) a naturalistic emphasis, (2) transaction and process, (3) multiple levels of analysis, and (4) ipsative–normative methods of study (Lazarus, 1981).

First, the naturalistic emphasis proposed well-designed field studies providing "ecological validity" (Lazarus, 1981). Observations in subjects' natural settings contradict laboratory analysis which can neither provide descriptive data, create a full range of stress–coping processes, provide adequate data over time, nor ethically subject people to real-life stressors. Further, Lazarus asserted that control over measurement, presumed in past positivistic research, may be an illusion, and that confounding variables may actually be valuable sources of data (Lazarus, 1981). This emphasis on naturalistic inquiry is not new or unique to Lazarus, as sociology and other disciplines have developed specific field methodologies (Schatzman & Strauss, 1973).

Secondly, transaction and process refer to the description of stress and coping as factors in a dynamic reciprocal process of interplay or transaction between the person and the environment. Research requires methods that observe change from moment to moment within transactions and across multiple stress–coping encounters.

The third tenet, multiple levels of analysis, proposes the analysis of stress and coping at interdependent social, psychological, and physiological levels. Mediators must be examined at all levels independently and interdependently. This tenet appears well suited to issues of family study. However, Lazarus has not elaborated on the family aspect.

Finally, the ipsative–normative methodology refers to respect for intraindividual perspective, as well as group, or interindividual responses. Ipsative refers to the many facets of the same person and how the person functions in a variety of contexts. Lazarus (1981) asserted that research can be both ipsative and normative at the same time. This approach may lead to a research design that relinquishes the large numbers of (normative) cases required for statistical significance in favor of "more intensive examination of the same persons across occasions or over time" (Lazarus, 1981, p. 191). Thus, the number of persons observed is reduced and the number of observations is increased for individual persons or families (Lazarus, 1981, 1984a, 1984b). This tenet is particularly relevant for the management of multiple family variables.

Integrating the Frameworks

To clarify the research to be discussed here, links among philosophies must be recognized. McCubbin and Patterson (1983) affirmed the important links between the physiological (Selye, 1974) and the psychological (Lazarus, 1966). Koop and Keating (1990) proposed a model that combines elements of family stress theorists (Hill, 1958; McCubbin & McCubbin, 1987; McCubbin & Patterson, 1983) and psychologists (Lazarus and Folkman, 1984). They proposed, as did Lazarus, that coping — as a process by which a family solves problems, accesses resources, manages, or otherwise manipulates variables of stressors, resources, or appraisal — is the central concept. Major factors in the hybrid model are (1) focus on appraisal and coping, (2) brevity and simplicity and (3) accounting for processes over time.

Other links in research literature that are less defined are those between the study of individuals and of family units. Menaghan (1983) outlined the differences between individual and family coping, along with associated conceptual and methodological implications. Boss (1988) suggested, from a general systems perspective, the merging of individual and family literature. Both individual and family group indicators are important in understanding children's stress–coping phenomena. Individual psychosocial symptoms are not purely intra-psychic, but represent and affect the family system. However, this approach must not overlook the idea that families are not simply the sum of the variables of individuals.

Similar to Koop and Keating, though not for identical reasons, I propose that family stress–coping research needs an integration of the ABCX model for families and the cognitive–transactional model for individuals. A complete theoretical model would also include the following criteria (Feetham, 1984, p. 8):

1. The interdependence among the individual and the family, the family system, and the environment
2. The environment defined as the natural environment and the human-built environment (Morrison, 1974)
3. The family or family system as a mediator between the individual and society

The work of Lazarus has largely been applied to individual adults, rather than families or individual children. Although Lazarus occasion-ally mentions the concept of "family," the cognitive–transactional model neither accommodates an adequate definition of family nor attempts to recognize the complexity of interacting variables charac-teristic of the concept of family, except as they affect the individual. The ABCX model embraces the concept of family, but methodological difficulties in identifying "family" variables and sources of data con-tinue.

The works of both Lazarus and McCubbin initiated a conceptual shift from the cross-sectional examination of stressors and reactions to an emphasis on the *process* of stress–coping situations. Lazarus's (1981) philosophy effectively enhances aspects of ABCX theory. It refines the possibility for adequate definition of concepts—particularly variables B (family resources) and C (perception)—with methodological implications.

Both the cognitive–transactional and the ABCX models recognize the interactive ability of coping processes to affect and be affected by stressor situations. For example, McCubbin and Patterson (1983) noted in the ABCX model, that some coping efforts may actually contribute to a greater pileup of strain from stress. Lazarus and Folkman (1984) observed that sources of stress emerge not only from the environment but also from "coping ineptitudes" (p. 313). Thus, both models acknowledge that while stressors provoke the coping response, they may also be outcomes of coping processes. Such dynamic views of stressors in family systems implies methodological complexity. Lazarus escapes the issue of such complexity by avoiding the family context.

The ABCX model has been generally applied to major life stresses, such as chronic illness of a family member, and the cognitive–transactional framework has recognized phenomena of daily life stress in healthy individuals: Neither has explained how well people persist in positive adaptation.

Lazarus presents variables of resources, or mediating variables, in a broader, less structured context than Hill or McCubbin. This view— that resources both intervene in many contexts and affect many factors of the stress–coping transaction—is a more realistic reflection of reality.

Furthermore, although McCubbin and associates (1980) clarified stress as "the interaction of a particular type of event with its perception" (p. 857), the concept of perception or appraisal has more significance in the cognitive–transactional model, which states that stressors can reciprocally affect and be affected by the individual and family.

Acknowledging both Hill's (1949) revised family stress theory and Lazarus's (1981) cognitive–transactional philosophy, along with the other frameworks discussed as backdrops for my current study, the perspective opens to include a larger universe of the family context, revealing questions left unanswered by traditional stress-adaptation or stress-events theories. The holistic, humanistic focus upon individual differences, and the significance of individual and family perception and appraisal over time, embraces and respects human nuances formerly excluded as confounding variables.

This approach offers a contrast to the remnants of traditional stimulus–response ideas of operant conditioning, particularly in work with children. Lazarus's emphasis on individual cognitive intrapsychic and appraisal factors, combined with Hill's attention to the family unit, allow for consideration of processes and events over time and the unique complexity of human beings. This framework reaches beyond more simplistic behavioral stress-management approaches.

Finally, combining these philosophies opens the arena for an examination of healthy or adaptive states as distinctive, allowing for the proposition that positive adaptation or health may be more than or different from the simple absence of pathology.

It must be noted here that adequate development and testing of such a hybrid model has not been done and needs to be further explored. Indeed, the integration I propose herein reflects only the conceptual foundation for an explorative study whose purpose was to empirically describe and refine concepts, without intending to test theory. However, I hope that this acknowledgment of philosophical influences, even in research that does not generate or test theory, will open perspectives in family research.

RESEARCH ON FAMILY STRESS AND COPING

An overview of family stress–coping research is difficult since it includes work in many disciplines. Families have been studied in sociology, psychology, family science and therapy, education, medicine, and nursing. A review of specific studies will not be presented here. However, I offer general observations on investigations of family stress and coping including the areas of family characteristics related to particular types of stressors, identification of family resources and coping patterns, and intervention to promote positive stress outcomes.

Family Characteristics and Particular Types of Stressors

Family stress is most often studied in terms of family characteristics and hardships related to particular stressors. Examples of such characteristics include communication patterns, family structure (Feetham, 1984), family resilience (Patterson, 1991), family types (Lavee & Olson, 1991), and family boundary ambiguity, as in the loss of a family member (Boss, 1980a, 1983, 1987).

Types of family stressors most often studied include what are often termed "normative" and "nonnormative" stressors. Traditionally, normative stressors have included predictable developmental transitions, such as the transition to parenthood. Many of these studies of stressors observe the advent of the first child. Few studies of the stressors of parenthood have examined the dynamics in families with many children. Other normative stressors include midlife adjustments of child rearing, occupational stress, and the entry of women into the workplace. Later life transitions include retirement, widowhood, and caregiving to elderly family members.

The nonnormative stressors most frequently studied include natural disasters, loss of family members, family violence, and chronic illness. Whereas it is widely accepted that children may be affected the most in the long term by such crises (Garmezy & Rutter, 1983), studies of families frequently do not include the young child's viewpoint, and studies of children are often done in isolation from the family context, such as in the school or therapy setting. One exception to this pattern is the significant work with the families of children with chronic or terminal illness. Generally, these efforts have focused on the physical and emotional hardships of the child, siblings, and parents (Holaday, 1989; Kazak & Marvin, 1984; McCubbin, 1989; Schilling, Schinke, & Kirkham, 1985; Walker, 1988).

Adams (1986) depicted stressors on a grid with permanent versus temporary stressors along one axis, and voluntary and involuntary stressors on the other. He described stressor variations as normative or nonnormative (expected or unexpected), internal or external to the family in origin, temporary or permanent (acute or chronic), voluntary or involuntary, and singular or compounded (clustered) with other stressors. The clustering of stressors (perhaps similar to the McCubbins' view of pileup) increases the probability of crisis. Adams also recognized the significant factor of the family perception of stressors.

The emphasis in many of these studies has been upon roles and role change (Feetham, 1984), usually from the viewpoint of marital adjustment or parental role adaptations, or role change and task realignment (Boss, 1980b, 1983; Mederer & Hill, 1983). Acquisition of roles is thought to be more stressful than role loss (George, 1980) and role strain greater with nonnormative stress than with normative stress (Boss, 1988; Pearlin & Lieberman, 1979). The dearth of research on role adjustments in young children and siblings is remarkable.

Perspective Taking

One rarely discussed aspect of role interaction is that of perspective taking. Most often studied in child development, perspective taking usually refers to a degree of cognitive development prerequisite to the development of moral reasoning (Walker, 1980). Walker outlined stages of perspective taking related to moral development. Definitions included "[a realization] that the self and the other can view each other as perspective-taking subjects," and "a realization that each self can consider the shared point of view of the generalized other" (p. 132).

Perspective taking is usually described as an ability in young children or marital partners to imaginatively put themselves in the place of another (Long, 1990). Perspective taking reflects empathic communication and concern, humanistic orientation, and emotional and communicative responsiveness.

Ruddick (1982) discussed the related concept of "maternal thinking," a quality of intellectual reflection, empathy, judgment, and emotion by which mothers attend to and connect with their own young children. By this quality, mothers are thought to take the perspective of the child while in the role of parent.

Although the study of perspective taking has been largely limited to child-to-other in the development of moral reasoning (Garrod, Beal, & Shin, 1990; Gollin & Sharps, 1987; Taylor, 1988), the construct (perhaps with a new conceptual and operational definition) holds promise as an important variable in the study of parent-to-child individual and family interactions in response to stress.

Family Resources and Coping

Resources are often the focus of explorations of family adaptation to stress. The personal resources most often studied include environmental and financial resources, education, health, and personality characteristics. Other family resources include decision-making and problem-solving abilities and processes, sense of control, social support, and coping patterns. Family strengths, such as adaptability, esteem, and health, need to be explored, as the inclusion of both stressors and strengths could be useful in empirical studies. A better understanding of family strengths might help to break the barriers of stereotyped expectations, as McCubbin (1989) noted in a comparison of single- and two-parent families. Whereas she noted lower financial and maternal coping and optimism scores in single-parent families, such families also exhibited greater adaptability. Furthermore, she reported no difference in stress levels, family types, esteem–communication, mastery and health, or extended family social support between one- and two-parent families.

Social support has received by far the most attention as an individual and family resource. There has been considerable discussion on the definition and role of social support in promoting positive stress outcomes. Some have measured social support as a dimension of family resources (Holroyd, 1974; McCubbin, Comeau, & Harkins, 1979; Schilling et al., 1984), while others have viewed social support as a part of coping (McCubbin, McCubbin, Cauble, & Nevin, 1979).

While there is general agreement that an understanding of effective family coping may be more important than a knowledge of the nature, frequency, or severity of family stress events, little work has been done in the area of coping, particularly at the level of the family unit. Most research in the area of coping has been done with individuals, drawing from the cognitive–phenomenological philosophy of Lazarus and Folkman (1984). McCubbin and colleagues (1980) suggested that individual coping behaviors within a family will (1) decrease vulnerability, (2) strengthen or maintain family resources, (3) reduce the hardships of stressor events, and (4) influence the environment by altering social circumstances. Such ideas seem to flow from cognitive–phenomenological coping theories, and further validate the need to merge family and individual theoretical literature.

Intervention to Promote Positive Stress Outcomes

In view of the need for more descriptive data regarding family responses to stress over time, especially the need to identify effective coping strategies, intervention studies seem necessarily limited. Most of these investigations have studied the effects of various types of social support or educational programs on families experiencing particular stressors, such as terminal illness or parenting risk factors (Aiken, 1982; Boss, 1988; Grobe, Ilstrup, & Ahmann, 1981). Lazarus and Folkman (1984) and Ryan (1988) asserted from different perspectives that such intervention studies, particularly some stress-management programs, may be premature in view of the need for knowledge of individual appraisal, including children's perceptions, positive family function, and effective coping responses.

METHODOLOGICAL TRENDS AND IMPLICATIONS

Integration of theoretical models and philosophies, of theory and research, and of research on family education and practice are profoundly complex. In-depth theoretical construction is useless without the application of appropriate methods for valid testing. Larzelere and Klein (1987) offer an extensive exploration of relevant methodological issues, and Adams (1988) reviewed the past and proposed future directions for family study.

Limitations of Traditional Methodological Trends

It is inadvisable to integrate theories unless links are evident in research and practice. As family science moves beyond positivism toward empirical explorations and applications, theory must become more explicit and useful in guiding research (Larsen & Olson, 1990; Lavee & Dollahite, 1991; Schumm, 1982). Lack of good scholarly communication among theorists, researchers, and practitioners pervades family theories and studies. This is aggravated by the fact that such an interchange encompasses several disciplines.

The complexity of the family unit, and the significance of both its entirety and its components, present concerns about both *what* should be measured and *how* data are best accessed (Gilliss, 1983; Larzelere & Klein, 1987; Olson, 1985). Family measurement has been an issue for decades (Straus, 1964). Trends in the study of family stress–coping phenomena have paralleled research trends in family research in general. First, with a few recent exceptions (Curran, 1983, 1985; McCubbin & Figley, 1983), there has been a propensity to focus on abnormal families or families dealing with particularly pathological or stressful conditions (Feetham, 1984). Knafl and Grace (1978) pointed out that data from problem families may not be generalizable to healthy families.

Regarding these studies, McCubbin et al. (1980) noted the following:

> This emphasis on the trying, and often times crippling, impact of child-related stressors has been helpful in sensitizing the researcher and clinician to the traumas of chronic and demanding human experience. However, only a handful of these investigations have attempted to shed light on the reasons why some families are better able than others to adjust and manage chronic, long-term stressors. (p. 860)

Exceptions to the traditional inclination toward the study of major crisis or pathology are included in a significant body of literature related to normative transitions of families, such as marital adjustment (Boss, 1980a), parenthood (Miller & Sollie, 1980), sibling rivalry, single- and step-parenting, work stress, retirement, and others referred to as "entrances and exits" by Paykel (1974) and Rutter (1983). Other views of positive variables are offered by the McCubbins in analyses of family resiliency and strengths (McCubbin & McCubbin, 1988).

One trend in family research has been the repeated analyses of large demographic data sets. Such large-scale surveys with increasingly sophisticated techniques for analysis are predicted to continue (Adams, 1988). These presentations are certainly helpful in identifying broad trends among large populations, but caution must be exercised in the use of such data as valid reflections of actual daily family life. Responsibility for valid interpretation increasingly falls to the investigator. A significant related example is the work of Olson and associates (1983). The study gave a battery of tests to 2,692 individuals. Although the sample did include 412 adolescents, no preschool or school-age children nor siblings were represented. Tests, written from the perspective of adults and completed by adults (with the adolescent exceptions) sought data about children, but not from children, significantly limiting the "family" perspective. Representation of family realities was further limited by an overriding husband–wife (couples') view of family variables. Problems of validity among such studies only become further compounded as subsequent ad hoc analyses presume that the data give authentic, reliable representations of families in general, such as is evident in Lavee and Olson's (1991) later analysis of the same data set.

A second trend in family research has been an overwhelming reliance on one family member, primarily the wife/mother, as the data source. The result has been an abundance of so-called family research that actually reflects one person's perception of family phenomena (Feetham, 1984; Olson, 1977; Thomas, 1987; Uphold & Strickland, 1989). Larson (1974) referred to this practice as the most significant methodological weakness in family research. Walters, Pittman, and Norrell (1984) pointed to a number of authors who acknowledged that an accurate picture of the family cannot be represented from either the report of a single member or a simple additive score from two or more members. Others have further observed that the family is not the simple average or sum of its members (Adams, 1988; Larzelere & Klein, 1987; White, 1984). Some scholars (White, 1984) have further described the "discrepancy between the sampling unit and the unit of analysis" (Walters et al., 1984, p. 498).

Beyond the issue of measurement of the family as a unit are the issues of relationships, interdependence, and reciprocity within the family. Jones (1987) noted that individual psychosocial symptoms are not purely intrapsychic, but represent and affect the family system. However, even when the purpose of the research is to examine relations or transactions within families, frequently the theoretical and data collection foundations are aimed at the individual (Fisher, 1982).

Although data are occasionally drawn from the marital couple or even from the husband/father, children's voices, from their own subjective perspectives, are rarely heard. For example, McCubbin et al. (1980) noted that "research on children's reactions to loss have tended to emphasize the children's sensitivity to their mother's reaction, rather than the children's involvement in personal grief" (p. 859). Other examples are the numerous recent works on family violence, which have not included the subjective view of the child. An interesting general pattern has been to report data from the mothers' perspective as *family* research, while reporting the less frequent observations from fathers' or children's viewpoints as research specific to those groups.

Most data on young children in a family context have been drawn from parents, teachers, and clinicians. Ryan (1988) observed that "most of what is known theoretically and empirically about stress and coping has been developed by adults for adults" (p. 1). Gochman (1985) further noted the need for family definition both from the view of parent–child influences but also between siblings, and for multilateral measurements. For example, a study of family stress, or even of stress in a particular family member, might draw data from parents, children, siblings, and perhaps even extended family members.

A third trend noted in family stress–coping research is the focus on cross-sectional, episodic time periods (McCubbin et al., 1980). Because so few longitudinal studies are performed, we know little about the nature of stressors or patterns of coping over time. Because coping strategies are not created in an instant, phenomenological observations are needed of families as they deal with life conditions as the family develops over time. Wright and Leahey (1987) asserted that issues of time and meaning are important links in family patterns of interaction and adaptation.

Instruments and Methods

One major factor contributing to the problem of appropriate family data sources seems to be the nature of research instruments. Most measurements of family functioning are paper and pencil tests seeking responses from an adult informant (see Epstein, Baldwin, & Bishop, 1983; Lasky et al., 1985; McCubbin et al., 1982; Olson et al., 1983, 1984; Pless & Satterwhite, 1973; Roberts & Feetham, 1982; Smilkstein, 1978). Occasionally adolescents are included as informants, but apparently not because of an interest in the adolescent perspective but rather because they are assumed to be at a sufficient level of cognitive development to complete adult-focused questionnaires with ease (see Oliveri & Reiss, 1982; Olson et al., 1983). Thomas and Barnard (1986) noted that ". . . paper and pencil tools do not truly measure family 'functioning' or family 'satisfaction': they measure the individual respondent's *perception* of the family. Any internal or external observer will have a unique perspective . . ." (p. 11).

That observation is particularly true in stress and coping instruments. As noted, the recent events lists are largely drawn from the adult perspective. Coping scales also generally reflect an individual's viewpoint of family behavior.

A few scholars have attempted to interpret data from observation of family interactions, or from entire family units, or to creatively combine individual scores to achieve family measurements (see Ball, McKenry, & Price-Bonham, 1983; Fisher, Kokes, Ransom, Phillips, & Rudd, 1985; Ford & Herrick, 1974; Godwin, 1985; Grotevant & Carlson, 1987; Lowman, 1980; Walters et al., 1984). Ransom, Fisher, Phillips, Kokes, and Weiss (1990) reviewed issues of individual and family measurement. However, most family measures continue to exclude the subjective viewpoint of the child. Though items on most commonly used instruments seek a family response, data are usually sought from the perspective of the traditional two-parent family, and forms are oriented toward an adult viewpoint, usually completed by a single adult member of the family.

A review of some frequently employed instruments indicates that whereas marital conditions are frequently addressed, young children's individual and sibling concerns and situations are largely absent as family variables (see Epstein et al., 1983; McCubbin et al., 1979; McCubbin, McCubbin, & Thompson, 1986, 1988; Pless & Satterwhite, 1973; Roberts & Feetham, 1982; Touliatos, Perlmutter, & Straus, 1990). Even when the study was child centered, data collection frequently avoided the child. While some may argue that a parent is able to reflect a child's viewpoint, this has not been scientifically validated. Indeed, some data may indicate the contrary (Knutson, 1991).

Certainly, the future may bring increased and improved use of methods such as observation by videotaping (Wiseman, 1981), projection techniques with sentence completion or art, specifically directed diary keeping, or perhaps the invention of multiple versions of instruments for use at various developmental levels. Increased multidisciplinary collaboration will be necessary for such complex ventures. Adams (1988) pointed out that most of the responsibility for the interpretation of empirical meaning in findings lies with the researcher, rather than the statistics.

Implications for Future Research

Past family research developed a foundation for explaining and predicting family stress responses. From this foundation, future works must include prescriptions for effective family stress management and coping. Current research seeks to define concepts of family stress, coping, and resources from the perspective of all family members.

One possible explanation for the lack of data from young children is concern about the reliability and validity of instruments directed at cognitively immature informants. The question of what age a child must be to provide usable data has not been answered. Certainly, traditional instrumentation will require some creative revision in order to accommodate data from preschool and school-age children. A perspective on family situations in which interactions among young children are considered as important as adult marital relationships may require some rethinking.

Future research will suggest effective interventions and the means for preventing illness and promoting positive adaptation. This can be done only by creating measurement techniques that accommodate individual and aggregate data, and by shifting the focus away from family dysfunction and toward the study of positive and effective family responses — away from pathology and toward a study of health. Methods of data analysis must manage both voluminous qualitative variables and multiple quantitative variables as the family equation expands. With the means to include all relevant variables, theory will thus expand to better reflect the reality of families in both illness and health.

SUMMARY AND CONCLUSIONS

Numerous theoretical perspectives from a number of disciplines are represented in family research. The multidisciplinary nature of family study and the complexity of factors involved provokes a need to draw from several frameworks for an integrated approach to analysis. Although the influence of several general theories has been great, the ABCX models of Hill and McCubbin combined with Lazarus's cognitive–transactional model have contributed most to the study to be described.

General research trends in family stress–coping phenomena were explored. These were analyzed in the domains of family characteristics and types of stressors, with particular attention to role interactions in normative and nonnormative stressors, dimensions of family resources and coping, and intervention studies. Methodological trends and issues for future research were reviewed, outlining the need for the creation of instruments that reflect multiple family viewpoints, especially those of minor children.

In family research, methods have mostly included paper–pencil tests, vast demographic surveys, or observations directed at adult members—usually the mother—of the family. The complexity of considering a collective family viewpoint has been avoided. Information about stress and coping in children has usually been *about* children, from the viewpoint of adults, rather than *from* children, reflecting their own subjective perspective. There is a need to develop measures that more accurately reflect the lived experience of all family members. Family scientists have begun to examine stress-coping concepts in their unique and complex application to the family unit. However, often the missing note in the harmonic chord of the family has been from the voice of the children. Thus, while volumes are written about husband–wife relationships in families or about how individual children cope with hospitalization, little is known about the child's view of stress and coping in the family context.

Stress, Coping, and Appraisal
among Children

Discussion of stress–coping phenomena among children in a family context elicits considerable conceptual, methodological, and empirical complexity. In research or practice with children, traditional methods and concepts are challenged.

One conceptual concern is the definition of "children." The term "children" may be applied to a familial–social position that may embrace individuals of all ages, including adults. When considering a comprehensive family context, such a sociophilosophical discussion of the term may be warranted. However, empirical considerations should dictate appropriate limits. Thus, the study to be reported here specifically defines children as school-age offspring of parents living together in a traditional nuclear family situation. Acknowledging the limitations of such a constrained empirical definition, but also taking "ordinary intact families" (Handel, 1985, p. 367) into account, the literature reviewed here includes the general category of minor children.

Another important methodological distinction is whether information is provided *about* children, regardless of who the informant is, or whether information is provided *by* children, regardless of its content. In either case there are implications for valid theory development, methodologies, and clinical validity. This distinction is not always clear in the literature.

In the past, research about children has overwhelmingly focused on stress and stressors, with less attention paid to the processes of appraisal or coping, particularly as empirically defined or validated by children themselves. However, the literature offers some direction for study. This chapter will review research on stress–coping phenomena among children and briefly explore the influence of mediating variables in the stress–coping process. This will be followed by notes on gender and a general discussion of method.

RESEARCH ON CHILDREN'S STRESS, COPING, AND APPRAISAL

Most of the work about children has focused on the individual rather than the family unit. Indeed, few studies of children have even included them within the context of a family setting.

Stress Measurement in Children

Stress measurement among children has generally followed adult models. Traditionally, the emphasis has been on major life events. However, there is some recent interest in children's daily hassles. Research on the subjective perspective of the child has included stressor lists that children rank according to perceived severity or threat and the development of inductive taxonomies of stressors derived from children's interviews, school class discussion, or sentence completion. Stress research in children will be reviewed according to those topics.

Major Life Events

As mentioned in Chapter 1, life events have been the traditional yardsticks for measuring stress among adults. Research among children has followed that model. Adult stress-events scales were first adapted to school-age children by Coddington in 1972. Coddington's instrument closely resembled the adult scale, listing parental death, divorce, and other adult events. Indeed, a comparison of Coddington's (1972) list and the adult list of Holmes and Rahe (1967) would indicate that perhaps the only stress events experienced by children were those experienced by the adults in their lives. Coddington's (1972) list is probably the best known and most widely used, but other similar scales have been proposed by Sandler and Block (1979), Elkind (1981), and Chandler (1981) who added school- and peer-related stressors.

Research among children has followed a long line of correlation studies associating stress events with illness or maladaptation, as noted in Chapter 1. Parental stress has been shown to be related to newborn health (Kirgis, Woolsey, & Sullivan, 1977). Child or family stress has been related to incidence of childhood respiratory tract illness (Boyce et al., 1977), asthma (Zlatich, Kenny, Sila, & Huang, 1982), disposition toward accidents (Knudson-Cooper & Leuchtag, 1982; Padilla, Rohsenow, & Bergman, 1976), migraine (Cooper, Bawden, Camfield, & Camfield, 1987), juvenile depression (Hudgens, 1974), and daily health changes in chronically ill children (Bedell, Giordani, Armour,

Tavormina, & Boll, 1977). Such studies among children are reviewed by Johnson (1986).

A similar approach has been to study the effects of family life events on child adjustment. Although ostensibly based on children's experience, the effects were actually rated by adults and usually evaluated by traditional adult measures of life events. Examples include works on cardiovascular disease risk factors (Hanson, Klesges, Eck, Cigrang, & Carle, 1990), social support, and problem solving (Dubow & Tisak, 1989; Dubow, Tisak, Causey, Hryshko, & Reid, 1991). Other examples include investigations of children's apparent adjustment to specific types of family adversity (Shaw & Emery, 1988) and to traumatic events such as parental divorce or normative stressors such as the advent of a new sibling in the family (McNamee, 1982).

Masten (1985) noted that correlations obtained in traditional life-events studies among children are usually quite low, though consistent. She proposed that the study of stress and coping in children must include a developmental perspective, including attention to age, gender, and cognitive and socioemotional maturity in the child's perception of stress. Invalidity based on developmental differences is a threat in methods that combine data from wide-ranging age groups of children.

Masten (1985) further described a proliferation of various life-events scales with insufficient data regarding their validity or reliability: "For example, a distressed parent of a . . . sick child may recall more negative events than a parent whose child is flourishing" (p. 546). Also, variables of life events confound with variables of symptoms, as it becomes unclear to what extent life events may be antecedent or the result of illness or maladjustment. Masten cited a need for research to focus on the influence of positive or negative mediating variables, such as social support, parental competence, and personal characteristics. Thus, the use of major life events as the operational definition in studies among children may be fraught with even more methodological and empirical difficulties than have been observed among adult studies. At the least, it seems that major life events may reflect only one aspect of childhood stress, and ought to be (1) validated from the child's viewpoint, and (2) perhaps combined with other measures for a more comprehensive definition of stress.

Daily Hassles

Among middle-aged adults, daily hassles have repeatedly been shown to be more strongly associated with somatic health than life events

(DeLongis et al., 1982; Kanner et al., 1981; Monroe, 1983). Ryan (1988) also argued that stressors identified by children appeared to be processes over time, perhaps resembling hassles, rather than the discrete events that typically appear on stress-events lists. Miller and associates (Miller, Tobacyk, & Wilcox, 1985; Miller, Wilcox, & Soper, 1985) tested hassles and uplifts in adolescents in two similar studies. In each study, they administered the hassles scale (Kanner et al., 1981) to thirty-eight 15- to 18-year-olds. One study sought a listing of experiences perceived as stressful and/or pleasurable. Findings, which supported other observations of adolescent stressors, were the following: concern about physical self, influence of peers, and worries about the future. The other study showed hassles to be negatively and significantly related to psychological and physical health, whereas uplifts were not significantly correlated to health measures. Colton (1985), Bobo, Gilchrist, Elmer, Snow, and Schinke (1986), and Compas, Davis, Forsythe, and Wagner (1987) developed similar hassles scales for adolescents. Each associated behavioral or reported relationship problems with high scores on negative daily stressors. DeMaio-Esteves (1990) reported that hassles were negatively related to perceived health status among adolescent girls.

Kanner, Harrison, and Wertlieb (1985) studied hassles and uplifts in 9- and 11-year-old children. Their work showed general self-worth negatively associated with hassles and positively associated with reported uplifts.

Another study (Kanner et al., 1991) tested 232 American sixth graders, using scales for hassles, uplifts, depression, restraint, friendship support, social competence, and self-worth. As expected, hassles were generally associated with poor outcomes—though more strongly by boys than girls—and uplifts were associated with more positive outcomes.

Concentrating on family structure, Kanner and associates (1991) compared subjects from intact, blended, and single-parent families and found that only the frequency of hassles differed among groups. On item analysis, children from intact families were less likely to report peer problems, feeling incompetent in school, and feeling bad when the teacher was upset with them. However, there were no differences on items dealing with the reported availability of parents.

Thus, daily hassles may be a promising approach to measuring what have traditionally been called normative stressors. There is a need for more empirical testing. There may also be a need to determine how hassles and major events fit together in stress measurement. Although there appears to be a current trend toward rejecting the life events approach, the concepts of both major and minor stressors certainly ought to be integrated.

Ranked Events

A few studies have attempted to rank children's perceptions of stressors. Yamamoto and associates (Yamamoto, 1979; Yamamoto & Byrnes, 1984; Yamamoto et al., 1987) asked school-age children to rank a list of major and minor stressors, developed by researchers in an attempt to examine day-to-day stress experiences. Ranked highest on the list were losing a parent, going blind, academic retainment, and wetting in class. Ranked *lowest* were a new baby sibling, giving a class report, going to a dentist, and losing in a game. Although the study has been criticized for the fact that children rated hypothetical stressors that they may never have actually experienced (Ryan, 1988), it still offers some insights. For example, whereas in the past family literature has affirmed that a new baby sibling is a normative stressor, this study suggests that validation must come directly from children before this is assumed.

Brown and Cowen (1988) compiled stressor lists from existing instruments and asked 503 school-age children to rate the degree of distress associated with specific stressors and whether they had actually experienced the stressors. Girls generally judged events to be more upsetting than did boys. The study affirmed the findings of Yamamoto and associates (1987) that children rated the "stressor" of the birth of a new sibling as the least upsetting, contrary to traditional adult-rated scales such as Coddington's (1972) list and other previous studies (Dunn, Kendrick, & MacNamee, 1981; Garmezy & Rutter, 1983).

Johnson (1989) found a simple frequency count of life events actually experienced by children to be the most significant predictor of children's responses to stress. School-age children in Brown and Cowen's (1988) study reported actually experiencing an average of seven listed stress events in their lifetimes. Such frequency counts in the context of pileup in family stress theory might also prove interesting.

Although stressor lists ranked by children move one step closer to a definition of stress from the child's perspective, there remain some issues of concern. First, most lists are derived by adults, usually researchers or clinicians. Thus the margins of error may widen in areas where (1) there may be some selective stressor items included that may not accurately reflect the child's view, or (2) other items that might reflect the child's perception may be inadvertently omitted from the lists. Second, since ranked lists contain a number of items that may not have actually been experienced by child subjects, the operational concept reflected by such lists may not be actual life stress at all, but rather anxiety or childhood fear. Furthermore, it is not clear whether children might rank actual life experience differently than hypothetical events.

Inductive Taxonomies

Several recent efforts to identify daily life stressors from the child's point of view have generated lists and taxonomies by inductive measures. Many of these were developed concurrently with, but isolated and separate from, the taxonomies to be discussed in my own study in Chapter 4.

Lewis, Siegel, and Lewis (1984) attempted to define a child's view of psychological distress in the development of the Feel Bad Scale. Through interview and small group discussion, they asked 50–60 children to respond to the question, "What happens that makes you feel bad, nervous, or worried?" (p. 117) Subsequently, 20 items were generated and tested among 2,400 fifth graders. Factor analysis revealed the three major stressor domains of (1) conflict with parents, (2) self-image and peer-group relations, and (3) geographic mobility. Only about one-fourth of the items reflected discrete events, while 14–15 items reflected role strains, or what might be termed cognitive-emotional stressors. Actually, the authors were not precise on the definition of "stressor," as they alluded to concepts of stress, anxiety, and a broad category of "feeling bad."

Though Lewis and colleagues (1984) specifically eliminated items related to physiological distress, Sharrer and Ryan-Wenger (1991) used the scale to demonstrate significantly higher stress scores among children with recurrent abdominal pain than children who did not report symptoms of stomachache.

Dickey and Henderson (1989) asked 141 school-age children, "When you are at school, what worries or upsets you?" Responses were classified into eight areas of stressors including, in descending order of frequency, school work, peer relations, personal injury or loss, loss of personal comfort, discipline, relations with teachers, family events, and miscellaneous.

Dise-Lewis (1988) also sought children's perceptions of major life events and hassles by verbal and written responses obtained directly from children through individual and group interview. Data were then tested in the form of a life-events scale. Events reflected the four major areas of (1) traumatic or crisis events, such as death of a parent, (2) common events, such as sports competitions, (3) role and relationship strains, such as arguments with parents, and (4) internal concerns, such as worries about self.

Explorations by Taylor (1980) and Dibrell and Yamamoto (1988) offered qualitative narrative data from informal interviews with children and parents. Taylor interviewed 25 healthy school-age siblings of children with chronic illnesses then described the effects on the well sibling of factors related to the ill child, and other intrapsychic factors related to the well child's own development. No a formal list of stressors was derived or frequencies among categories recorded.

Dibrell and Yamamoto (1988) interviewed 46 well children, aged 4–10 years, in small groups. Children were asked to describe situations that made them "sad," "worried," "upset," or "angry" (p. 15). The narrative reported responses of physical harm, parental sanctions, and peer relations. Fears and anxiety sources also included being lost or abandoned, hospitalization and medical procedures, and conflicts between parents.

Atkins (1991) reviewed 14 studies of stress and coping from children's perspectives. Two investigations sought data from children in interviews at home (Taylor, 1980; Walker, 1988). All other settings were school classrooms or hospitals. Five studies were of children as medical patients, two were of siblings of chronically ill children, and seven were of well children. Ten of the investigations employed interviews with children, from which four identified inductive categories of stressor coping lists (Dibrell & Yamamoto, 1988; Ryan, 1989; Taylor, 1980; Walker, 1988). However, problems with Atkin's review included a lack of distinction between studies of children with special problems and well children, and between stressor lists and coping taxonomies. There is a need for a more comprehensive and precise review of inductive studies.

These studies and those in Atkins's (1991) review are attempts to begin to identify and define stressors from the child's point of view. It would also be helpful to combine, compare, and test stressor and coping taxonomies that are now emerging. Although valuable, instrument development based on a single taxonomy, as some have attempted (Dise-Lewis, 1988; Lewis et al., 1984; Ryan-Wenger, 1990), may be premature.

Coping Measures among Children

The characteristics of coping continue to undergo scholarly scrutiny. Coping may refer to strategies or styles, or may be substituted for another concept altogether, such as stress management. However, the literature to date generally presents coping as responses to specific types of stressors. Therefore, coping will be presented here according to reports of children's dealing with major life trauma and daily life stressors. Afterward, inductive studies that identify coping responses will be explored, followed by a review of coping instruments for children.

Most research on children's coping has focused on responses to major traumatic events, such as illness, hospitalization, or personal disaster, like divorce of parents or death or illness in family members. There has also been considerable study of children's responses to the more normative stressors of daily life. Coping measures will be reviewed here according to those topics and attempts at instrument development will also be explored. It must be noted that though there has been significant assessment of children's coping responses (Zeitlin, 1980), the concepts of strategies, efforts, or styles have not been precisely clarified. Thus coping will be viewed here as the general realm of responses to stress experiences.

Coping with Illness or Hospitalization

A major area of study has been children's experiences with illness or hospitalization (Caty, Ellerton, & Ritchie, 1984; Zastowny, Kirschenbaum, & Meng, 1986). Dibrell and Yamamoto (1988) devoted an entire fear/stressor category, based on children's interviews, to "the world of people in white" (p. 18). The area of child responses to hospitalization and medical procedures has offered a common, convenient source of data. From it, coping strategies and styles have been identified (Field, Alpert, Vega-Lahr, Goldstein, & Perry, 1988; LaMontagne, 1984; Savedra & Tesler, 1981), the influences of moderating variables such as gender, health status (Bossert, 1990), temperament, and maternal behavior (Lumley, Abeles, Melamed, Pistone, & Johnson, 1990) have been examined, and various interventions have been explored (LaMontagne, 1987; Wolfer & Visintainer, 1975, 1979). Peterson's (1989) review of a few of such efforts noted several enduring conceptual and methodological concerns, such as the developmental dynamics of children, the need for attention to individual differences, and the temporally and situationally specific nature of coping processes. Dibrell and Yamamoto (1988) also emphasized the strong influence of the quality of the parent–child relationship.

Caty and colleagues (1984) attempted to identify and categorize coping patterns in an analysis of 39 case studies of hospitalized children, aged 20 months to 10 years. Using a descriptive methodology of content analysis, the authors identified 2,572 units of coping behaviors. These were categorized according to three major factors: (1) Information Exchange, (2) Action/Inaction, and (3) Intrapsychic influences. These factors were then subcategorized according to the age groups of toddler, preschooler, and school-age child. Information Exchange behaviors included information seeking, information limiting, and information giving. The Action/Inaction category included mastery, controlling, tension-reducing, self-protection, and self-comforting behaviors. It also included the behaviors of soliciting assistance, expressing emotion, and decision making. The third category of Intrapsychic characteristics, included behaviors and mental processes regulating emotion, such as denial or intellectualization.

The work on children's responses to health care procedures and hospitalization is important. However, generalization to other life situations may be limited. The extent to which coping responses of sick children are similar, or as effective, in other stressor situations is not known.

Coping with Major Trauma

Traditionally, coping research among children has focused on responses of special populations experiencing major personal trauma and painful situations, such as bereavement and loss (Brown et al., 1986; Furman, 1983; Masten, 1985), parental conflict and divorce, or abuse. Other works focusing on child populations at risk include analyses of the adaptation of siblings or families of chronically ill children (Drotar & Crawford, 1985; Holroyd & Guthrie, 1986). In this group are the studies of coping in siblings of children with chronic illness, including cancer. These were reviewed by Walker (1986).

There is a growing body of knowledge on the effects of overwhelming personal trauma on children. Whether experience with disaster toughens and steels a child or sensitizes the child to anxiety, thus becoming a burden in personality development (Terr, 1979), is a controversial question (Anthony, 1991).

A classic is the work of Garmezy and Rutter, best known for studies of stress and resilience in children suffering serious trauma. In 1983, they assembled researchers and clinicians to explore data and issues related to stress, coping, and pathology in children. Major stressors, such as war, death, divorce, poverty, and minor though traumatic stressors, such as separation from parents, were analysed in children from infancy through adolescence. Of particular significance was the emphasis upon developmental aspects and the implications of stress–coping phenomena in children. Although the focus was generally on childhood psychopathology, the effort presented provocative research questions about the nature of coping and resilience in children, suggested by a number of investigators from a number of theoretical perspectives.

Garmezy (1991) and others have noted resilience, competence, and creative coping among some children experiencing severe life stress. The source and role of such mediators must still be investigated. Indeed, there is much still to be learned about children's responses and needs in major trauma. However, the purpose of this study is to explore daily life stress among apparently well children. Therefore, major trauma among children will not be further explored here.

Well Children Coping with Daily Life

Among the first and most extensive works related to stress, coping, and adaptational processes in well children was the longitudinal study by Murphy and Moriarty, published in 1976. The exploration provided multiple psychometric data on 32 children over a period of 15 years. Measurements included various psychological tests, behavioral observations, and coping and vulnerability inventories. The multiplicity of data from a complex constellation of methods and observers provided for abundant discussion with implications for coping research. The study resulted in the Comprehensive Coping Inventory. Though the list offered important data related to childhood coping, it is impractical for general use as an instrument, since it includes 999 complex measures and variables.

In a preliminary report of the study, Murphy (1974) identified two major coping styles as (1) the capacity to "deal with the opportunities, frustrations, obstacles of the environment," and (2) "the capacity to maintain internal equilibrium" (pp. 77–78). Caty and coauthors (1984) later found Murphy's two broad classifications of internal and external coping to be inadequate. Furthermore, Murphy's data, while emphasizing the process, were interpreted largely from a psychometric orientation, rather than from current, more holistic theoretical frameworks.

The research offered questions appropriate to the rationale for my own study. Murphy and Moriarty (1976) studied, from a process viewpoint, a sample population of normal, mostly healthy children, focusing on the paucity of scientific data dealing with "the maintenance of normality" (p. 5). They further proposed that the difference between disturbed or unhealthy children and normal children was not the presence or absence of stress, but rather how problems were managed, revealing a need for exploration of coping strategies. Their investigation was one of the few seeking to identify coping patterns in children "who managed to stay 'normal' " (Murphy & Moriarty, 1976, p. 5).

Family, developmental, and education literature have devoted considerable energy to the study of how children deal with normative stressors, such as entering school, change of the family residence, or the advent of a new sibling. However, because adult researchers, teachers, and clinicians have created the existing lists of "normative" stressors of childhood, the validity of the resulting coping explorations may be in question.

Inductive Measures

Recently, several researchers have attempted to inductively classify school-age children's coping efforts from data drawn directly from children. Compas, Malcarne, and Fondacaro (1988) explored coping strategies actually used and the capacity to generate alternative solutions for coping in interpersonal and academic stress situations among children aged 10 to 14 years. They found that children used both problem- and emotion-focused coping strategies in response to both interpersonal and academic stressors.

Walker (1988) studied well siblings of children with cancer. Although she observed a particularly stressed group, the results contributed to the study of coping patterns among relatively well children. Following the cognitive–phenomenological approach of Folkman and Lazarus, she studied 26 siblings, aged 7 to 11 years, of children with cancer. Data included family demographics and coping patterns of siblings from the perspective of both parents and children. Data were collected by interviews conducted twice over a period of 3–10 days.

By analysing content, coping patterns were identified. Modifying Folkman's (1979; Folkman & Lazarus, 1980) approach, which identified emotion-focused and problem-focused categories, Walker used the two major categories of emotion-focused and behavior-focused, although she expressed difficulty with strict dichotomous assignment. From these categories, Walker identified three domains—intrapsychic, interpersonal, and intellectual—and subsequently several themes and subcategories. Unlike Taylor's (1980) review of stressors among siblings of children with chronic illness, Walker's taxonomy is focused less on the ill sibling, and thus appears to be more generalizable to well children.

Band and Weisz (1988) adapted Folkman and Lazarus's (1985) Ways of Coping checklist for use with children to observe the nature of the reported coping responses of school-age children. They found that in 96% of all descriptions children reported active coping, and in 3.5% of cases children responded by relinquishing control.

Ryan (1989) asked one hundred and three 8- to 12-year-old children to list coping strategies used to deal with given stressors. The results produced 13 types of coping efforts, including use of social support, avoidant activities, distracting activities, and cognitive activities.

The inductive studies described here represent a trend toward developing coping lists and taxonomies from qualitative data from children. Whereas methods of data collection and analysis have differed slightly, most of these taxonomies have been derived from a cognitive–transactional framework. The trend seems to emerge specifically from the disciplines of psychology and nursing. A specific multidisciplinary analysis of children's coping taxonomies as they are developing would be useful. Further, such data ought to be validated by all family members, and examined from a family framework.

Coping Instruments

A few attempts have been made to develop instruments for the measurement of coping in children. Boyd and Johnson (1981) published the Analysis of Coping Style, a picture-interpretation test marketed as a cognitive–behavioral approach to coping assessment in school-age children and adolescents. Although the theoretical framework of the instrument appears internally consistent, adequate reliability has not been established. Other major problems with the test seem to be its development based on data from teachers and clinicians rather than from children themselves, its testing of children with behavioral problems, and its emphasis upon forced negative responses.

The Coping Health Inventory for Children (Austin, Patterson, & Huberty, 1991) was developed to assess coping behaviors of school-age, chronically ill children. The instrument examines five conceptual areas of coping: competence and optimism, withdrawal, irritability and acting out, compliance with treatment, and seeking support. Whereas the test exhibits internal consistency and stable reliability, it elicits responses only from parents and not from the children themselves, and its use is limited to a relatively small, albeit important, subgroup of children.

Dise-Lewis (1988) developed the Life Events and Coping Inventory for 12- to 14-year-old children. The instrument assesses life events, both major and minor, and coping strategies. Items were generated from verbal and written responses obtained directly from 681 children by interview, with several stages of refinement and reliability testing directly. The extent of general use of the tool is unknown.

Elwood (1987), Wertlieb, Weigel, and Feldstein (1987), and Ryan-Wenger (1990) each developed coping instruments for use with school-age children, using a cognitive–transactional model. In all three cases, items were generated directly from children. Elwood interviewed 85 children individually and in school class discussions, seeking reports of actual stressors experienced and coping responses. Her work resulted in a major event inventory, daily hassle inventory, and coping response inventory for children of several different school grades, with fairly good reports on validity and reliability.

Wertlieb and associates (1987) tested a semistructured interview instrument, called the Child Stress Inventory, on 176 children. Coping responses were coded as Self, when coping behavior is directed at personal action or subjective distress; Environment, when behavior is directed at situations or people other than self; and Other when the child was "rescued" by another person.

Ryan-Wenger (1990) generated a list of coping responses by individual questionnaire and school group discussion among 103 school-age children. The most common responses were then analyzed by experts and pilot tested as a coping instrument. The tool was then tested on 107 children. Validity and reliability measures were impressive. However, it must be acknowledged that items were drawn from presentation of hypothetical stressor situations, rather than stressors actually experienced by the children (Ryan, 1989).

Among the most widely used measures for children's coping behavior is Zeitlin's (1985) Coping Inventory. The test is completed by an adult who rates the child according to effectiveness of particularly adaptive behaviors. Coping with self (personal needs) and the environment (external demands) are rated. Children's coping styles are measured as productive, active, or flexible. Forms of the test are available for preschool and school-age children.

A notable attempt at measurement of coping of the entire family is the F-COPES, designed by McCubbin et al. (1982) to identify family coping strategies. While construct validity and reliability have been tested, the test is limited to problem-solving approaches and behaviors, and does not address individual cognitive coping responses. Thus, it fails to address the developmental implications and individual coping dynamics of children.

The psychometric value of many of the instruments described must be acknowledged. However, in view of the growing, yet still limited, data related to children and coping (especially from the viewpoint of the child), development of an instrument for general use must wait for the collection of prerequisite descriptive data. There is much work to be done to refine concepts, such as coping efforts, strategies, or styles. Furthermore, as in the case of stressor lists for children, more data would be helpful for a multidisciplinary comparison, integration, and testing of the inductively derived coping taxonomies.

Regarding the stress–coping process in children, the major research question remains: What is it? Thus, it seems most useful to continue a factor-isolating approach, using qualitative, inductive methods, given the present state of the science.

Appraisal

There is considerable recent multidisciplinary interest in cognition, perception, perspective taking, and individual meaning from the child's point of view (Cox, 1991). It is becoming increasingly evident that data from parents, teachers, or clinicians may not accurately represent the child's world view. For example, in a study relating stressful events to divorce, Wolchick, Sandler, Braver, and Fogas (1986) compared ratings of parents, clinicians, and children. Whereas rank orders were correlated, assigned stress values as perceived by the children were notably different from those assigned by parents and clinicians, substantiating the significance of individual perception of appraisal, and the need for measures sensitive to children's perceptions.

Other studies that have compared the ratings of parents, clinicians, and children have demonstrated significant differences between adults' and children's perceptions (Ryan, 1988; Wolchick, Sandler, et al., 1986; Yamamoto & Felsenthal, 1982). A recent, increasing number of studies have sought children's own appraisals and coping reports in particular chronic stressor situations. For example, Grey, Cameron, and Thurber (1991) studied 103 children with diabetes, reporting that preadolescent and adolescent children coped differently, and that preadolescents were less depressed, less anxious, and coped with chronic illness in more positive ways than adolescents.

Barnes (1988) studied 64 depressed and nondepressed school-age children, finding that depressed children reported more negative life events and daily hassles, and were more likely to use avoidance and emotional discharge to cope with stressful situations than nondepressed children.

Even in the use of life-events scales, appraisal becomes an important variable. In her study of 264 seventh-grade children, Call (1983) demonstrated the significance of the mediating variable of individual appraisal or perception, suggesting that, particularly among children, individual perception is more significant statistically and clinically than scores on stress-events scales. Dise-Lewis's (1984) study further underscored the importance of the variable of individual perception in children by noting that children who have experienced particular stress events recently perceive them as more stressful than those events experienced in the past.

The significance of individual appraisal and the tenet of naturalistic emphasis have been reinforced by a few studies of stressors in childhood that have obtained data directly from children by innovative methods. For example, Pidgeon (1981) conceptually classified the spontaneous questions asked by hospitalized preschool children to determine the function of the questions in relation to coping. Implications for specific intervention methods were then drawn from an analysis of the needs expressed by the children through their questions. Bryant (1985) further sought data regarding children's perceptions of their sources of support by observations he made during and following a neighborhood walk.

Assessment of appraisal in children presents a research challenge because of the necessity of children's expression of thoughts, perceptions, and emotions. However, such innovative techniques as those described above, or others, such as imagery (Siegel, 1986) or drawings (Siegel, 1986; Sturner, Rothbaum, Visintainer, & Wolfer, 1980) may offer helpful data. One study (Sturner et al., 1980), among hospitalized children, examined children's drawings of a human figure before and after the children experienced a venipuncture procedure. The drawings were interpreted according to emotional or anxiety indicators. Such a method, with valid interpretations of "psychological meaning" (Sturner et al., 1980, p. 330), could help circumvent the communication challenges presented by children of varying linguistic and cognitive abilities.

Interventions

Several intervention programs in stress management are offered for children (Elias et al., 1986; Englehardt, 1986; Hendricks & Wills,

1975; LaMontagne et al., 1985; Richardson, Beall, & Jessup, 1983). McNamee's (1982) work presented a broad spectrum of childhood stressors that ranged from normative school and sibling stressors to divorce and death experiences. Considerable work has been done to reduce the stress of hospitalization, medical procedures, and psychological loss (LaMontagne, 1987; Meng & Zastowny, 1982; Poster, 1983; Wolfer & Visintainer, 1975, 1979). Hunsberger, Love, and Byrne (1984) and Caty et al. (1984) reviewed such studies among children.

Most stress management interventions for children follow age-adjusted adult models of relaxation, biofeedback, guided imagery, and other educational modes, with little validation from children themselves. Most are derived from a clinical information background rather than from empirical testing, and are promoted in lay literature (Chandler, 1985; Saunders & Remsberg, 1984; Youngs, 1985). Indeed, a review of child stress-management programs leaves the reader with a marked impression that they may actually be aimed at management of parental stress *about* their children.

Testing of interventions often employs dependent variables that are indirect reflections of momentary stress, such as heart rate, blood pressure, relaxation, or sense of well-being. Thus, the enduring effects of interventions on daily life stress or relationships remain to be discovered. The relation of interventions to other aspects of coping or their implications for children's development are also unknown.

MEDIATING VARIABLES IN CHILD STRESS-COPING PHENOMENA

Mediating variables are viewed here as events, people, or personal characteristics that mediate or buffer stressor effects, enhance coping efforts, or offer coping resources (Sorensen, 1991). Among children, some of the same variables commonly studied in adults are important, particularly social support (Dubow et al., 1989, 1991) and locus of control (LaMontagne, 1984; Rothbaum et al., 1979).

Though the significance of social support in children's stress-coping responses cannot be denied, little is known about children's perceptions of the meaning of social support. For example, we do not know how, by whom, and when it is most helpful in the life of a child. The study reported in Chapter 4 will illustrate another point, which is that there may be a difference in the social support that must be actively sought by a child and the social support that is available, offered by parents, teachers, or siblings, for example.

Usually, such variables are studied individually as they are associated with adaptation to stress. Using semistructured journals, I have begun a taxonomy of mediating variables, studied as a group, from the viewpoint of children (Sorensen, 1991). Major themes include sources of emotional comfort, physical–social activities, physical comfort, and social support.

Of all aspects of stress–coping phenomena in children, research in the area of mediating variables seems least likely to follow traditional adult-based models, particularly in the area of personal characteristics. Examples include the works on child resilience, vulnerability, and temperament.

There is increasing recent interest in the concept of resilience or invulnerability among children experiencing stress (Anthony & Cohler, 1987; Felner, 1984; Murphy & Moriarty, 1976; Werner & Smith, 1982). Garmezy (1991) defined the complex construct of resilience as "the tendency to rebound or recoil, to spring back, the power of recovery" (p. 463). He further described characteristic factors of resilience including individual factors, such as temperament, cognitive skills, responsiveness to others, etc; familial factors, such as warmth, cohesion, caring parents, etc; and support factors of meaningful social support outside the family. Resilience has also been related to children's control beliefs (Wannon, 1990) and intelligence (Rutter, 1983).

Such resilience has been described among chronically ill children (Sinnema, 1991) and their siblings (Leonard, 1991). Patterson (1991) described characteristics of family resilience when a child is chronically ill. Such characteristics included balancing the illness with other family needs, maintaining clear family boundaries, competence in communication, attributing positive meaning, flexibility, commitment, active coping efforts, and maintaining positive social relationships.

On the other hand, vulnerability is a recognized variable about which little is known. Rutter (1983) debated whether stress events caused emotional or mental illness, or the presence of such disorders or their precursors render the individual (or family) more prone to stressful life experiences. The question remains whether vulnerability to stress is a condition of poor or inadequate coping resources, or a particular complex characteristic of some individuals in spite of resources, or both. Felner (1984) explored factors related to childhood vulnerability. Essential elements of the concept remain to be examined.

Temperament is another complex personal construct that seems to be a significant mediator in the stress–coping process. Rutter (1982) defined temperament as the "preponderant style in how an individual does things or *how* he or she responds to people and to situations, rather than to *what* the individual does, or to *why* he or she does it, or to the behavioral capacities or abilities that he or she manifests" (p. 1). Thus, temperament seems to be an abstraction rather than an observable behavior. Aspects of temperament include emotionality, activity level, and sociability (Dollahite & Winterhoff, 1992; Goldsmith et al., 1987; Rutter, 1987). Dollahite and Winterhoff (1992) described temperament as a "filter or amplifier" by which perceptions, stressors, and resources are mediated.

The study of temperament has been focused on observations of infants and young children (Kagan, 1983; Garmezy and Rutter, 1983). There is increasing study in the relationship between children's temperament and various aspects of stress and family relationships (Dunn & Kendrick, 1982; Kyrios & Prior, 1990; Stevenson-Hinde & Simpson, 1982; Thomas & Chess, 1977).

There is a need for more study of children's temperament in relation to (1) response to stressor events (Rutter, 1983), (2) patterns of change in temperament with age, and developmental effects on coping responses, and (3) the reciprocal nature of interpersonal interactions in relation to differing temperaments of individuals within families and effects upon family stress–coping phenomena. There is some evidence that temperament may influence sibling and parent–child relationships, which might affect the nature of social support within families during stressor situations.

Dollahite and Winterhoff (1992) expanded the concept to include family temperament. They described the variable in the context of a resource management model of family crisis–stress, identifying eight different individual and family temperament styles. Although the theoretical basis for family temperament still needs to be tested, it offers promise as an example of an effective multidisciplinary integration of concepts related to individual and family stress.

Another important mediating influence in the lives of school-age children is that of sibling relationships. Handel (1985) noted the dearth of attention to the sibling subsystem of families, especially in view of the volumes contributed on marital couple and parent–child relationships. Generally, in stress–coping studies where data were drawn from children themselves, sibling influences, either positive or negative, were listed by many children.

Citing and comparing two of the major works on sibling relationships (Irish, 1964; Schvaneveldt & Ihinger, 1979), Handel (1985) outlined special issues in sibling relationships. These included equity related to performance and application of rules, resolution of disputes, and handling scarce materials within the family; maturity in power and knowledge; loyalty, related to availability to each other, sharing, handling family information, and protection; and individuality, related to privacy and self-demarcation.

A few others (Dunn, 1985; Powell & Ogle, 1985) have outlined the intensity and social significance of sibling relationships to the normally developing child, as well as to children with special developmental and/or illness needs. Much of the work on stress–coping and siblings has been focused on siblings of chronically ill or terminally ill children. These studies are reviewed by Drotar and Crawford (1985) and Walker (1986).

In considering the stress and coping of childhood, particularly from the view of the culture of childhood, sibling concerns offer significant mediating variables as sources of stress, in perception or appraisal, and especially in coping. Obviously, sibling relationships comprise a unique source of social support. Even the simple contrast of the parallel (or not so parallel) sibling relationships within the family have obvious potential influence on stress–coping phenomena. Closer observation of children as they move between distance and intimacy, resolution and conflict in the context of sibling relationships is needed. It is an important area in child stress–coping research.

Given the dependent role of the child within the family, it would seem that mediating variables from the context of the family would also be especially important to the positive adaptation of the child. There is a need to explore such issues as parental competence, family roles, and socioeconomic conditions from the viewpoint of resources. However, these will not be discussed here.

The list of potential mediating variables in stress–coping phenomena among children is long, and a fertile field for exploration. No attempt at an exhaustive list is made here. My purpose is simply to point out an important area of study.

GENDER

One important mediating variable in children's stress and coping is that of gender. Scott (1986) defined gender as "a constitutive element of social relationship based on perceived differences between the sexes" (p. 1067). The gender dichotomy has been identified as a mediating variable in much social science research. Though some have studied gender from the viewpoint of persistent maladaptive social habits and processes that seem to construct and maintain gender-related differences (Bem, 1983; Ferree, 1990), this work will simply identify the gender differences among children that emerge in specific stress–coping phenomena.

Joffe (1973) and Thorne (1986) demonstrated that children themselves actively adopt gender-related behaviors, symbols, and characteristics in play and relationships. Most inductive studies of stress and coping in children have uncovered spontaneous gender role differences or other descriptive differences between boys and girls.

As the study of stress–coping in children evolves, it is important to recognize and clinically accommodate gender differences. For example, though boys and girls do not differ in number of hassles, there is evidence that they are experienced differently. Kanner and associates (1991) observed that girls reported the following hassle events to be more "potent," or significantly worse, than did boys: parents fighting, sibling interference, not liking appearance, teasing, losing something, parental concerns, not knowing the answer in school, feeling inferior to other children, and not enough privacy.

The nature of social support among children offers interesting gender implications. Bryant (1985) found that girls benefitted from more intensive, intimate social involvements, while boys sought more extensive, casual relationships. Similarly, Waldrop and Halverson (1975) observed that, among children from ages 2 to 7, quality of relationships and social skills among peers seemed related to *numbers* of friendships among boys, whereas among girls such variables were more related to *intensity* and *intimacy* of peer relationships.

In addition, Ryan (1989) noted in her inductive list of school-age children's coping strategies that boys named significantly more physical activities whereas girls reported more emotional responses and social support seeking behaviors. Wertlieb and associates (1987) also reported that school-age girls were more likely to describe support-seeking coping responses, whereas boys reported coping in a more individualistic or self-oriented way.

Such thematic differences bear closer analysis. At least taking note of gender differences in studies of children seems an important methodological detail, whether or not that is the primary purpose of the research.

METHODS

Looking forward to the study to be outlined in the next chapter, it is important to understand the author's interpretive framework in relation to epistemological and methodological issues. Therefore, I now offer some general notes on methods. More specific methodological reports related to the study will be presented in Chapter 4.

Research related to stress and coping in adults, families, and children has traditionally followed the predominant normative, quantitative approach. The positivistic orientation has generated knowledge by providing statistically supported relationships among quantitatively cast variables. Deductive data have been drawn largely from scales, quantitatively reduced surveys, or quasi-laboratory approaches that attempt to control variables and show correlations or to isolate particular adaptive responses in order to test theory.

On the other hand, there is a growing trend toward widening the philosophical and methodological lens by which concepts are qualitatively examined, offering research "motivated by curiosity [rather than] by theory" (Handel, 1985, p. 368). The term "phenomenology" refers generally to a qualitative approach to study, attributed to the existential philosophies of Husserl, Heidegger, and Sartre, as well as to a specific methodological approach. It is used here in a broad descriptive sense. The purpose of phenomenological research is to describe a phenomenon, not usually to generate theories or models (Field & Morse, 1985), but rather to see "the patient as he really is, knowing him in his own reality" as opposed to "seeing merely a projection of . . . theories about him" (Roche, 1973, p. 3).

Phenomenology addresses the source of the data, rather than theories about the data, in search of meaning. Cohen (1987) further explained that the concern of phenomenology is

> with individuals and their view. Informants, not theories, are consulted and trusted. Also important is studying the *Lebenswelt*, the world of everyday lived experience: individuals are studied in their natural context, not in contrived situations. The natural attitude, the everyday unreflected attitude of naive belief, is studied with phenomenologic methods. (p. 31)

Valid stress–coping research is currently performed according to both quantitative and qualitative philosophies.

In dealing with child subjects, there may be an epistemological and theoretical need to expand the perspective of "ways of knowing." Just as some (Belenky, Clinchy, Goldberger, & Tarule, 1986) have explored women's ways of knowing, a similar epistemological expansion to expose children's ways of knowing might prove helpful. Indeed, subsequent integration of such viewpoints in family study would enrich the family perspective.

Current theories already established in child study might also be expanded and their concepts redefined. For example, most developmental theory on children was not derived to include situations of illness, loss, or other stress such as hospitalization. Subsequently, child behavior during illness, which may well be developmentally normal and effective under the circumstances, has often been termed regressive according to normative developmental theory. Thus, the 10-year-old child who denies, cries, reverts to an imaginary companion, or indulges in physical self-comforting behaviors during hospitalization may be exhibiting effective coping strategies. An expanded epistemological view of children's ways of knowing might allow a redefinition of development based on circumstance.

Epistemologies and Definition of Concepts

As mentioned in Chapter 1, a definition of concepts and constructs has been particularly elusive in stress–coping research. Limited methods may have contributed to this problem. Dennis (1986) noted that by purely quantitative methods, "hypotheses are derived and scales developed to measure the constructs; scales often become the operational definition of the constructs themselves" (p. 8), which explains some of the methodological difficulties mentioned in previous chapters that perpetuate a trait, rather than process, orientation in stress–coping research. Examples include the frequent use of anxiety scales, Type A–B behavior scales, stress-events scales, or simple muscle tension as measurements of stress.

Often, given the ambiguity in attempts to define stress, the scales themselves have become definitions for stress. Coping can then become a loosely defined measure of adaptation, whereas valid information is needed on coping patterns and repertoires. Inductively derived data might also contribute to greater precision in definition of such other significant factors, such as vulnerability or resilience.

Jones (1983) argued that from a qualitative interpretive perspective, "concepts and theories become essentially exploratory instruments that have no epistemological priority over the phenomena of the social world" (p. 151). Jones further pointed out that when the participant researcher brings theories and interpretive schemes to the study situation, definitions and outcomes are influenced them. Ultimately the adequacy of a theory is dependent upon its accurate reflection of reality from the viewpoint of those who live inside that reality.

The Significance of Individual Differences

To effectively address the stress–coping transaction, methodologies must accommodate individual differences as significant mediators in the natural setting. Until recently, factors such as individual differences or other qualitative characteristics have been set aside without study, or even ignored as confounding variables, though Rutter (1983) noted the "striking" effect of individual differences in studies of children's responses to stress. Dennis (1986) further noted:

> In classic measurement theory where the observed score is equal to the true score plus error, the idiosyncrasies, uniqueness, and individualities that may seem unrelated to the concept being measured yet influence each person's responses are relegated to the error term. Likewise in an experimental design, the subjectivity of the individual and uniqueness which makes him or her different from others in the same treatment group becomes the within-group mean square error term. Ironically, it is the most intriguing and the most elucidating of the phenomena in question. To improve the possibility of finding the significance they seek, however, investigators attempt to reduce the error terms, thereby suppressing the richness of spontaneous differences among persons. (p. 8)

Data are needed from those people who respond differently from the statistical majority (Lazarus, 1981), and there is a need to open the focus, for example, to promote analysis of healthy populations in their natural settings.

Naturalistic Settings and Subjective Report

Several scholars affirm the need for data collection directly from the naturalistic perspective of subjects by self-report. Although acknowledging the problem of method variance, or "the dilemma that how one measures a phenomenon affects the content of the observed variance and the findings of the research" in self-report data, Lazarus and Folkman (1984, p. 321) affirmed subjective report to be the "primary source" of data in stress–coping research. Indeed, they urged the use of such subjective data to "identify meaningful relationships." They reasoned that ipsative, naturalistic, self-report data are primary to building theory that may subsequently support other convergent methodological techniques, such as physiological and behavioral observations whose present use in stress–coping research may be "premature" (p. 327).

Acknowledging that research which successfully employs qualitative methods is dependent upon valid, first-hand, subjective accounts, the researcher who seeks authentic subjective data directly from child informants encounters some unique challenges. Among these are developmental immaturity in cognition and language; differences in world views, life experience, and daily activities; and barriers stemming from a common perception children have of adults as authority figures. Such challenges have occasionally precluded adequate, specific methods.

Unfortunately, theoretical assumptions regarding the validity of self-report and the necessity of the subjective viewpoint in qualitative research are often side-stepped for expediency in collecting data about children. With few exceptions in child and family studies (Amato & Ochiltree, 1987), validity is sometimes overlooked based on the premise that, due to social, cognitive, or linguistic immaturity, children are unable to competently interpret or to offer meaningful descriptions of their world.

Yamamoto and others (1987) have recognized and described "the culture of childhood," which is unique from the world of adults and ought to be considered in working with children:

> For two people who have lived side by side for such a long time, the adult and the child appear to know amazingly little about each other! On the seeming assumption that they sufficiently understand children and/or that the young do not know themselves well enough, adults continue to speak for children. An upshot of this general orientation has been the relative lack of information on how the world actually appears to youngsters themselves. (p. 855)

Subjective, descriptive data, in addition to objective information, are needed to provide meaning and direction for supporting successful adaptation to stress. For example, Mullan (1983) noted that even in the use of life-events scales, reliable data are best drawn from personal interview.

In research among children, limited data have been obtained from the children (subjects) themselves, particularly from within a family context. For example, both Coddington (1972) and Chandler (1981) developed widely accepted instruments for measuring stress events in children from data gathered from mental health professionals and teachers, without validation by children. Cohen (1985) questioned the validity of using only measures of parental report, in her own study of siblings with cancer. She recommended data collection directly from child subjects where possible.

Family Context and Longitudinal Data

Although traditional viewpoints have offered significant information, reductionist methods have sometimes overlooked the holistic nature of stress–coping phenomena, particularly in children and families. There is also a need to consider children in family contexts in research and clinical practice (Combrinck-Graham, 1988). Descriptive data are needed for methods that provide meaning and direction to supporting successful adaptation to stress within a family context. In family research, methods must somehow draw data from all members and allow for a view of the family constellation over time.

Furthermore, longitudinal data are needed to accurately reflect the phenomena of daily life. There is some evidence that reports of stress–coping variables are most accurate when the stress and coping processes actually occur, rather than as recollections of past experiences or as projections based on hypothetical events. This is especially true in children.

There is some evidence that, over time, school-age children provide stable survey responses to factual questions, but lower stability on items seeking opinions (Holaday, Turner-Henson, & Swan, 1991). Amato and Ochiltree (1987) also reported that responses from children are most valid "if researchers stick to the here-and-now" (p. 674).

One-shot, or even repeated-measures, designs may not accurately reflect the processes of day-to-day human experience, particularly in the areas of stress and coping. Instead of trying to achieve stability in repeated-measures or cross-sectional designs, we must find ways to collect and interpret data over time in ways that include a valid child's viewpoint. The invention of methods, such as structured or directed diaries that would allow children to report the here-and-now at consecutive points over time, may be effective.

It would be useful to harness the surge of current, multidisciplinary interest in qualitative methods for collaboration in dealing with children. Collaborative methods might include work using action research methods, interpretive interactionism, life history methods, cognitive mapping, dramatization, art, theatrical metaphor, and so on.

Specific Methods: Diaries and Others

The validity of qualitative data is dependent upon authenticity, and best obtained by unobtrusive measures. The tradition among unobtrusive instruments in the social sciences has been the use of interviews, questionnaires, and observation. Denzin (1973) explored other creative unobtrusive means, such as public documents, physical traces, and observations.

Deatrick and Faux (1991) outlined pediatric qualitative methods such as interview, play involvement, semistructured tools like sentence completion, diaries, and drawings. They discussed solutions to the unique challenges of working with children, related mostly to the vast differences between child informants and adult investigators in cognitive development, physical maturity, and social status.

One little-used method for gaining naturalistic subjective data over time is the diary or journal (Sorensen, 1989). Emerson reportedly urged Thoreau, "Record your own spontaneous thought and you will record that which men everywhere find true for them also" (Haight, 1942, p. ix); and Baldwin (1977) noted, "The journal is a connection of the self with the self" (p. xiv). Journal studies exist in history and the humanities, mainly as descriptions of memoirs (Jenson, 1983).

Similarly, life history and case study methods were used extensively in sociology in the 1930s and 1940s, but apparently fell into disfavor during the last few decades due to the emphasis on positivistic empirical measurement (Denzin, 1973). Sociologists have recently shown renewed interest in the study of personal documents and life history methods (Bertaux, 1981; Denzin, 1983). Jones (1983) described the life history method as follows:

> [It is] a unique tool through which to examine and analyze the subjective experience of individuals and their constructions of the social world. Of all research methods, it perhaps comes closest to allowing the researcher access to how individuals create and portray the social world surrounding them. The life history methodology offers an interpretive framework through which the meaning of human experience is revealed in personal accounts, in a way that gives priority to individual explanations of actions rather than to methods that filter and sort responses into predetermined conceptual categories. (p. 147)

Journal keeping has advantages similar to those of life history methods. A few studies in education have employed purposive journal keeping for data collection (DeWine, 1977; Foorman, 1974). Steeves and Bostian (1982) cautioned that there may be significant, unique socioeconomic and educational characteristics in subjects willing to participate in diary studies and also noted low response rates and powerful subject resistance in diary studies. The literature is limited regarding the use of journals in health-related areas, except in therapy or education. Diaries are generally used in health research as a means to record daily changes in physical symptoms or emotional states (Butz & Alexander, 1991; Rakowski, Julius, Hickey, Verbrugge, & Halter, 1988; Robbins & Tanck, 1982). The technique has been used with adults, and to observe children by parental report. Similar works have been done in women's health (Woods, 1987).

A few works with diaries among children also exist. Manning, Manning, and Hughes (1987) analyzed open-narrative diaries recorded by 20 first-grade children over one school year. They found a wide variety of content that fell into 10 broad categories. It was interesting to note that one category included pictures only, where children communicated the daily entry with original art. Buxton (1982) also reported the value of school-age children's journals in assessing development.

In a family context, it seems that use of diaries could provide simultaneous data from several family members and allow data collection over time in a naturalistic setting. Diaries are common in therapy, sometimes as open-ended, spontaneous documents for personal insight, sometimes semistructured in the form of checklists of symptoms, feelings, interpersonal events, and so forth. Diary use for research, though less common, seems to be a reasonable method for collecting descriptive data.

Combined Quantitative–Qualitative Approaches

Although it is tempting to embrace phenomenological methods and qualitative data exuberantly, caution must be exercised so as to retain the strengths of meaningful quantification and objectivity. Further caution is warranted to avoid practicing either research method solely based on habit or trend. Rather, the selected methodological approach ought to reflect the most appropriate means to answer research questions, accurately analyze data, and promote valid clinical interventions.

Traditionally, some disciplines such as psychology have pursued a quantitative experimental orientation, whereas others like sociology or social anthropology have promoted qualitative designs. There is an argument for combining traditional quantitative approaches with qualitative methods. Sandelowski (1986) suggested that qualitative methodology combines scientific objectivity with artistic integrity, as "the researcher communicates the richness and diversity of human experience in an engaging and even poetic manner" (p. 29). Qualitative methods emphasize the meaningfulness of the research, whereas quantitative methods provide control.

Bargagliotti and Trygstad (1987) further proposed combining quantitative and qualitative methodologies in the study of stress and coping. Their work compared the findings of qualitative and quantitative studies, which revealed that quantitative methods identified discrete sources of stress, and qualitative methods described coping processes over time. The comparison showed the strengths of both types of methods.

As noted in Chapter 2, there is interest among some scholars in integrating theoretical frameworks across disciplines. For example, theories from psychology about the individual, from sociology about the family, and from human development about the child each offer specific models, concepts, and languages for definition. The integration of models, with a resulting clarification of concepts, may move theories toward a better representation of empirical reality. Just as the movement toward multidisciplinary theory integration, responsible integration of methods and designs also seems in order. As such integrations and combinations continue — accompanied by the necessary rigor and precision — we will come closer to concept definition and meaningful interventions.

The investigation to be described here did not advocate or test particular methodological definitions, philosophies, or theories. Indeed, the discrete differentiation of one qualitative design from another has yet to be clarified in methodological literature (Brink, 1987). The purpose of this study was rather to seek — by the most reasonable, valid and reliable methods, according to the state of current knowledge and theoretical background — the answers to the research questions.

In view of the purpose of the study, and in view of the practice of qualitative researchers to "do what works" (Swanson-Kauffman, 1986, p. 61), a combined quantitative–qualitative descriptive strategy was employed. I recognized current theories as philosophical points of reference and "exploratory instruments" (Jones, 1983). Phenomenology and grounded theory methods suggested a means for data collection and provided a general context for the goal of describing the stress–coping experience in children. In addition, quantitative descriptive methods allowed for data management and reduction.

SUMMARY AND CONCLUSIONS

Research using traditional stress-events measures has mainly focused on the maladaptive effects of isolated or additive traumatic events, and has frequently overlooked individual appraisal and coping, especially from the perspective of the child. Hassles lists, although derived by adults, hold some promise as more valid stress measures. In recent studies where stressor lists were generated or rated by the children themselves, (1) the study setting has nearly always been outside the family, in schools or health care agencies, and (2) the children may not have actually experienced the stressors that they are asked to respond to or rank. Thus, stressor scales may fall short of the full spectrum of stressors actually experienced by children, particularly in the family context.

Although conceptual definitions of coping among children remain ambiguous, scholars have made recent strides in identifying coping phenomena, particularly in relation to major life trauma, and illness and hospitalization. Coping with more common, daily life stress has also begun to be identified from the child's view by a few inductive taxonomies of children's coping responses. Several objective coping instruments have also recently been developed, although it appears that more valid tools might be developed after analytic integration of existing taxonomies.

There is increasing acknowledgment of the concept of appraisal among children. To accommodate children's perceptions in research, creative methods beyond traditional paper–pencil tests or interviews need to be employed. Valid inductive data from the viewpoint of the child must precede valid intervention development, although a few stress-management interventions have been proposed. However, many such programs (1) are modeled on adult-based programs, (2) lack empirical validation over time, and (3) seem inappropriately popularized among lay literature.

Several important mediating variables in stress–coping phenomena among children include social support, sense of control, resilience, temperament, sibling relationships, and gender. The area of intervening factors in children is a virtually unexplored field of study.

In order to address issues in children's stress and coping adequately, methods must be expanded. I propose the integration and combination of quantitative and qualitative philosophies.

Despite the problems noted, the recent progress in the study of stress and coping among children has been remarkable. Works that have sought data directly from children and scholarly inductive taxonomies begin to lay a firm foundation for further validation and theory building.

An Exploration of Children's Stressors and Coping Responses

Data increasingly suggest that stressors, individual appraisal, and the coping responses of daily life are the most accurate predictors of health or illness. Currently, there exist few valid measures of these variables among children. There is limited knowledge about the degree of stress experienced by children, no means to predict the risk to stressors, and few valid prescriptions for prevention or management. Prerequisite to valid measurement or intervention development, stress–coping processes among children must be identified and described.

Using a combined qualitative–quantitative descriptive method, this study attempted to refine a conceptual taxonomy of day-to-day stressors, coping efforts, and coping resources drawn from 42 well children, 7 to 11 years of age. Coping variables were cognitive, emotional, and behavioral responses to reported stressors.

Coping resources were viewed as actions, thoughts, people, events, situations, or things reported by the children to prevent, buffer, or mediate stressor effects, assist in coping efforts, or enhance well-being, revealed by responses to the daily question, "The best part of today was . . ." The resources that emerged resembled "uplifts" more closely (Kanner et al., 1981) than the traditional resources described in the environmental or material sense.

ASSUMPTIONS

In view of the nature of qualitative inquiry, which presumes that the researcher is the instrument, and in view of the fact that the assumption of value-free inquiry is currently challenged even in positivistic study (Guba, 1981; Reason & Rowan, 1981), I recognize and acknowledge my own idiosyncratic values, beliefs, and assumptions associated with this study.

Observation of Children

In this study, I ascribed to the basic beliefs regarding children as subjects as described by Walker (1986):

> Underlying all professional interaction with children is a respect for the unique perspective of the individual child. Respect for the child is enhanced by attempting to understand each individual child's world view. Genuine respect requires the professional to strive for nonjudgmental interactions. (p. 29)

I also assumed that children of the age group observed were capable and willing to comply with individual data collection over time; that children generally respond openly and honestly — as best they are able from their personal life perspective, whatever that may be — when afforded an appropriate vehicle, and the basic respect described; that healthy children possess a potential interest in personal challenge, growth, and discovery regarding themselves; and that children are appropriate informants in specific aspects of family research.

Children, like adults, respond from both a personal and family environment. Children are an important component of the entire family context. Walker (1986) noted that:

> Interaction with children is also influenced by the belief that all children possess the potential for unlimited . . . psychosocial growth. Although credence is given to theories of human growth and development . . . children can, and often do, exceed the age limitations described in growth and development theories . . . children (may) exceed the expectations for their age with regard to moral development (Kohlberg, 1968) and cognitive development (Piaget, 1952). . . .
>
> Children are sensitive to and influenced by parents' attitudes, beliefs, and values, but do not automatically mimic those attitudes, beliefs, and values. Children are capable of processing available information and arriving at conclusions with a perspective different from parents'. Based on this assumption . . . data on the *child's* world is best obtained *directly* from the child rather than *indirectly* through the eyes of the parents. (pp. 29-30)

Such assumptions allowed me to enter the adventure of discovering children's world views.

Theory and Methodology

To repeat Kaplan's (1964) admonition, "no human perception is immaculate. . . . We always know something already, and this knowledge is intimately involved in what we come to know next" (p. 131–133). Thus, several of the theoretical philosophies listed in Chapter 2 influenced the direction of this study.

As noted, qualitative methodological philosophies generally preclude the existence of particular presupposed theoretical frameworks. Although this investigation followed a qualitative descriptive design, current family stress and cognitive–transactional theories (as discussed in previous chapters) contributed to the philosophical and methodological orientation from which the rationale, purpose, and methods of the study evolved. This study emerges from a theoretical orientation, but specific, adequately developed, theoretical frameworks related to stress–coping phenomena in children do not yet exist. Therefore the purpose of the investigation was not to test theory, but rather to contribute to a foundation for concept definition and refinement, and thus to subsequent theory building and testing.

The aim of the research was description and conceptualization rather than hypothesis testing. However, though data were descriptive, they were not totally narrative. Frequencies among identified domains and categories were calculated, and percentages among groups were compared to enrich the new knowledge base. Data were gathered from the children and parents directly, from written daily journals. The original research on 32 children also included a sentence completion instrument, which has been described (Sorensen, 1990). Data from that method will not be explored here. Further data were gathered through children's spontaneous drawings.

INFORMANTS

Subjects were drawn from volunteers from suburban areas of five western states. Families were recruited by response to letters describing the study that were sent home with elementary school children. Ten additional children entered the project. Five were selected for pilot study, and not included in the final analysis. Five other subjects eventually withdrew from the study by not completing at least seven daily journal entries. Follow-up of these families revealed that the journal-keeping experience was perceived as either too long or too inconvenient.

The study sample included 42 subjects, 17 boys and 25 girls, and both parents, from 30 families. The age range of the children was 7 to 11 years, with a mean age of 9.27 years. The children were healthy (determined by health history and scoring within normal ranges for all components of the Child Behavior Checklist by Achenbach and Edelbrock, 1981), lived with both parents, and attended public elementary school.

Family size ranged from one to eight children, with a mean family size of 3.52 children. The average age of the parents was 33.27 years for mothers and 37.88 for fathers. The parents were well educated (mothers with a mean of 2.17 years of college and fathers with a mean of 3.22 years). All fathers were employed, and 40% ($n = 12$) of the mothers were employed outside the home.

Selection of the school-age group was based upon tenets of developmental theory. According to Piaget (1952), the child in the stage of concrete operations (age 7–11 years) has evolved logical thought processes, has shed some of the egocentrism of earlier stages, and has become more social. Internalized cognitive activities have also developed to a point of effective social communication. Kohlberg (1964) noted that the child of this age has begun to acquire a sense of moral order, authority, and fair play. Erickson (1963) observed that social development and involvement in the school culture are crucial to a child of this age. Thus, school-age children would be expected to be able to express themselves about stress–coping phenomena to an adequate extent, and would not be expected to be submerged in the more egocentric tasks of identity evident in children just younger or older. Indeed, Band and Weisz (1988) demonstrated that children as young as 6 years are aware and able to articulate daily life stressors and coping responses, and can even evaluate the efficacy of their own coping.

METHODS

Instrument Development

A panel of academic and practice "experts" developed the initial diary instrument. These experts included three members of the faculty of a university college of nursing, two members of the faculty of a university college of health, one educational psychologist, one child psychologist in practice at a children's hospital, one counseling psychologist in private practice, and one pediatric nurse practitioner.

A sentence completion list (adapted from Walker, 1986) was used to elicit children's reports of coping responses to specific hypothetical stressors. Data from a group of children using that instrument are reported elsewhere (Sorensen, 1990). Expert consultation was followed by a pilot study of instruments with "field experts": five families completed diaries for 1 week. To test items and terms intended to elicit children's reports of stress, coping, and resources, as conceptually defined for the study, the following items were included in the daily semistructured journals:

1. What bothered me most today . . .
2. This is what I did about it . . .
3. What helped me most today . . .
4. The best part of today was . . .
5. The worst part of today was . . .
6. Sometimes I worry about . . .
7. This is what I do about it . . .
8. This is what helps me not to worry . . .

The most significant observation from the pilot testing was the apparent ineffectiveness of the term "worry" in eliciting children's reports of stressors. Though Dickey and Henderson (1989) and Lewis and colleagues (1984) included the term "worry" in seeking children's views of sources of stress, the term seemed difficult for children in this study to interpret, evoked the fewest stressor reports, and did not seem effective in eliciting actual sources of daily stress. The instrument was revised to remove the word "worry" and adopt "upset," which better elicited a child's description of the degree and nature of stress, without biasing responses toward particular emotions produced by such words as "sad," "angry," "afraid," "happy," and so forth.

Originally, there was some concern that a child's response to the item, "this is what I did about it [the reported stressor] . . ." would provide only behavioral responses, when cognitive, emotional, in-trapsychic data were also desired. However, as noted in assumptions about children discussed previously, children seemed to instinctively understand that the item sought the coping response of the child to the specific stressors listed. As results indicate, children readily reported intrapsychic and behavioral responses.

The pilot families, parents and children, commented on the unnecessary length of the journals. So it was reduced to the following three simple, open-ended statements, followed by the option of a drawing: (1) "This is what upset me today . . . ," (2) "This is what I did about it . . . ," (3) "The best part of today was. . . ." Each child was given an identical set of 12 colored markers for optional drawings.

The journals were completed individually by parents and children over a period of 6 weeks. Parents were instructed to complete the daily journals as if answering for the child (item example: "This is what upset my child today . . ."). Thus the open-ended measure sought a subjective report, and allowed and encouraged individual differences to emerge.

Validity and reliability were of primary importance, although not in the traditional positivistic sense. Drew (1986) argued that "in phenomenologic research the recounting of past experience is regarded as reliable data insofar as it is an expression of the feelings, thoughts, and emotions involved in the phenomenon being described" (p. 41). Colaizzi (1978) further suggested that validity in qualitative analysis must be measured with its own purpose as the standard, that is, that data are valid to the extent that they actually describe the subjects' experience of phenomena.

The content and construct validity of the semistructured journals were enhanced by the following factors: (1) data were retrieved directly from at least two members of each family: one child and one parent, (2) data were collected over time, and (3) data frequency was recorded among identified categories, enriching the perspective. Such validity and reliability were further strengthened by the critical analysis of the instruments by the panel of experts, followed by the pilot study.

Procedures

An appointment was made to meet the families. All sessions, except three, took place in the subjects' homes. During the session, procedures were explained, informed consent obtained, and the demographic questionnaire with health history and the Child Behavior Checklist (Achenbach & Edelbrock, 1981) were completed by the attending parent, which was usually the mother. The written health history and Child Behavior Checklist were used only as screening tools to assure that the children were generally physically and emotionally healthy.

Children and parents were given the semistructured daily journals in six packets of seven journals (one for each day for 6 weeks), with the following instructions: (1) parents were to respond to journal items as they perceived the child might answer, without consulting the child; either or both parents could complete the parent's journal, indicating who was the informant in the appropriate space on the form, (2) parents were not to coach the child on his or her journal as to content or grammatical form, although they could remind the child to complete entries, (3) if the child or parent was not willing or able to make a journal entry, blank forms were to be submitted for those days in which entries were not made. Indeed, to reduce testing as a possible source of stress, families were told that entries were not required every day. Families were instructed to return one set of journals from the child and parent weekly in the postage-paid envelopes provided, regardless of how many entries were made for the week.

The children required remarkably little explanation or instruction. Few children asked questions. Most children seemed to intuitively understand the open-ended items of the journal.

Analysis

Data were submitted to content analysis, an inductive taxonomization process of identifying the categories and patterns that emerge from naturalistic observation of variables. The parent journals were analyzed later and independently from children's journals, using categories derived from children's responses as a framework. All coding was done by the investigator, and all observations from all items of the instrument were coded in the taxonomy.

The reliability of coding was ensured by recoding randomly selected samples of data after a 3-month interval by the same investigator, and by simultaneous coding by another investigator. Investigator recoding agreement was .92, and coinvestigator agreement was .89. No further reliability determinations of the content analysis process were done.

Garvin, Kennedy, and Cissna (1987) noted that health-related problems are frequently best addressed by such categorization of phenomena. Their cautions regarding reliability in such analysis were considered. These warnings included the need for unitizing reliability, or consistency in category identification across judges and/or time (Folger, Hewes, & Poole, 1984). Such reliability is increased by the identification of small, concrete units and by the exhaustive coding of all possible observations (Garvin et al., 1987).

Because data were collected over time, frequencies per subject among categories were also recorded. Frequencies were then changed to percentages to allow for comparisons among girls, boys, and parents.

It must be noted that frequencies are offered only to enhance the description. The frequencies in any given category reflect a range from none to several possible responses from any one child or parent. Thus, the use of inferential statistics is not appropriate, since the assumptions of independent groups are violated. There is a temptation to presume evidence of statistical significance, and some scholars have attempted inferential approaches in similar situations (e.g., Ryan, 1989). How-

ever, these qualitative data must be accepted for their descriptive value
and face validity, and frequencies should be viewed as descriptive
"proportions," not the traditional mathematical units.

Positivists might discard the frequency figures as being without
value because they may not be plugged into accepted formulae,
whereas phenomenologists might discard the same frequencies because
they attempt to quantify the "lived experience." This is one of the
challenges of attempting to widen the positivistic view to include a
phenomenological viewpoint. I accept the challenge, and offer the
figures as one possible approach to obtaining useful information on the
proportions over time of actual responses from children and parents.
Others (Krippendorff, 1980) have proposed such quantitative applications to summarize qualitative data. Certainly frequencies and percentages among categories provide valuable information not given by the
simple "category saturation," which has become the standard in qualitative content analysis.

RESULTS

The total number of daily journal responses from children was 1,236,
ranging from 7 to 42 per subject. Of these responses, 477 (mean of
28.06 per subject) were from boys, and 759 (mean of 30.35 per subject)
were from girls.

The total number of parents' journal entries was 1,157, ranging
from 3 to 42 per parent, with 78 (6.64%) from seven different fathers
and the remainder from mothers. The mean number parental response
per subject was 27.54, or 6.42% less than the mean submitted by the
children.

The option was included in the children's journals to make a daily
drawing with the colored markers provided. The total number of
drawings was 616. The total number of drawings from boys was 267,
which represented a range of 0–35 drawings and a mean number of
15.71 per boy. The total number of drawings from girls was 349,
reflecting a range of 0–42 per girl and a mean of 13.96. The drawings
are discussed in Chapter 5.

CHILDREN'S DAILY STRESSORS

Content analysis of the data from the children's journals revealed 16
specific categories of daily stressors, within the domains of situations,

TABLE 1. Children's Daily Stressors

Domain	Category	Children (%)	Girls (%)	Boys (%)	Parents (%)
Situation	School	13.59	10.86	16.32	13.17
	Home chores	8.06	3.37	12.64	8.19
	Interruption	2.22	1.92	2.52	1.42
	Organizational demands	1.99	1.17	2.81	4.98
	Environmental discomfort	1.94	0.93	2.94	1.42
	Health care visits	1.16	1.26	1.06	0.71
	Subtotal	28.96	19.51	38.29	29.89
Self	Disappointment	10.65	16.31	4.99	17.44
	Physical symptoms	9.12	9.42	8.81	12.81
	Cognitive–emotional discomforts	7.43	6.52	8.34	5.34
	Personal responsibility	3.03	4.13	1.93	6.76
	Subtotal	30.23	36.38	24.07	42.35
Others	Friends	15.29	17.97	12.60	4.63
	Siblings	11.30	12.49	10.11	9.25
	Parental demands	5.43	4.34	6.52	12.10
	Family concerns	3.09	3.77	2.38	0.36
	School teacher	2.89	3.54	2.23	1.42
	Family members	2.81	2.00	3.61	0.00
	Subtotal	40.81	44.11	37.45	27.76
	TOTAL[a]	100.00	100.00	99.81	100.00

Note. Adapted from Sorensen (in press-a).
[a]All totals not equal to 100.00 due to rounding error.

self, and others. These categories and domains reflect refinements of concepts from data already reported (Sorensen, in press-a, in press-b). The domains are similar to the coping themes of self, environment, and other, identified by Wertlieb and colleagues (1987). Subsequent analysis of parent journals produced 15 of the same categories. Categories of stressors listing parent and child frequency comparisons are shown in Table 1. Descriptions of the domains and categories, with categories listed in order of children's reported frequency, follow.

Stressors from Situations

The situational domain included stressors whose source was in the events and situations of daily life.

The category "school" included reported stressors of the school atmosphere in general, as well as homework, tests, school projects, special assignments, and particular school subjects. The school subject most frequently mentioned as a source of stress by children was physical education, while the subjects most frequently mentioned by parents were science and mathematics. The major type of stress in this category seemed to reflect required behavior related to school, over which the child had no choice or control.

"Home chores" were known, predictable tasks over which the child seemed to have no choice or control, and/or for which he or she reported a general distaste. Among these were babysitting, practicing the piano, cleaning the bedroom, etc.

"Interruption" represented the annoying, unpredictable interruption of plans or ongoing activities. These included situations where television choices or viewing were interrupted, or when the child had to come in from play, stop an ongoing activity to read, do an assigned task, or go someplace.

"Organizational demands" included time or task demands of scouting, sports, dancing lessons, etc.

"Environmental discomfort" included annoyances such as weather conditions or particular foods.

"Health care visits" to the dentist or physician were listed by several children as a source of stress, whether for well check-ups or illness.

Stressors from Responses within the Self

This domain included those categories of internally focused stressors perceived as threats, losses, challenges, or annoyances to intrapsychic equilibrium.

"Disappointment," or deprivation of a particular desire or plan, was a category that included apparent internal threats to the child's plans, desires, and hopes, and also disappointments in personal performance. Examples included not getting a part in a program, losing a ball game, not being able to play with a friend, a sense of personal loss at not performing well in a particular school subject, not getting the expected grade, or not doing as well as hoped in baseball or football.

"Physical symptoms" included injuries, illness, or other physical complaints such as fatigue or hunger.

"Cognitive–emotional discomforts" included specific fears, such as being left alone, feelings of lack of control (as when the family car broke down), concerns about family finances, and a sense of injustice (as when the child got in trouble for something actually done by a sibling, or was required to do a chore perceived to be unjust). Also included here were reports of unidentifiable unrest, ambiguity, or boredom. The source of stress was described as being from a center of emotion or inner feeling source, rather than from the environmental situations related to the stressor.

"Personal responsibility" indicated stressors that focused on the child's sense of disappointment in self. It included tardiness or forgetting things, such as assignments, homework, or chores. It also included losing or breaking objects (several children mentioned the stress of spilling liquids at dinner), where the context seemed to be an insult to a sense of personal responsibility. Another example listed by a few children was the sense of personal responsibility to score in a losing ball game.

Stressors from Others

Although interpersonal relationships may be perceived by some as environmental factors, this study interpreted relationships as a unique category.

"Friends" was the category listed most by the children. Responses included descriptions of the bothersome behavior of friends, as well as concerns in the relationship, such as "they're having fun, and I'm not," or "they think I'm a baby."

"Siblings" were reported by both children and parents as a significant source of stress, though not to the degree indicated in traditional developmental literature.

"Parental demands" were the stressors of required tasks or being in trouble with parents. These included punishments for unacceptable behavior (such as being sent to one's room), or the parent being upset with the child.

"Family concerns" included worries about a sibling, parent, or grandparent. The center of stress seemed to be concern about the relationships. It was remarkable to note that although there was a depth of feeling reflected in some of these responses from the children, parents seemed largely unaware of such stressors. Frequently, the children's concerns were directed toward an absent family member, such as an older sibling or father working out of town.

"School teacher" was listed by both children and parents as a source of stress. This category was coded separately from the category of school because the responses reflected stressors grounded in the relationship with the teacher.

"Family members" other than siblings included grandparents or cousins. This category was not noted among parental responses.

"No Stressor" Responses

In the pilot study, concerns were raised from parents that children might respond with "no stressor" or "nothing," when parents perceived that children may actually have experienced a stressor. This was validated by Dise-Lewis (1984), who found that memory and the perceived severity of stressors were more dependent upon time distance among children than among parents.

In frequency calculations, if the item in the journal related to stressors was left blank, it was simply considered missing. However, if the child or parent actually wrote words like "nothing," it was recorded as no stressor. Thirty-nine children indicated "no stressor" a total of 379 times (30.66% of all responses), with a range of 1 to 37 and mean of 9.72 among those children, or a mean of 9.02 when accounting for all children.

Thirty-three parents listed "no stressor" a total of 266 times (22.99% of all parental responses), with a range of 1–34 among 33 parents, representing a mean of 8.06 among those parent couples, and 6.33 per total parent sets. Thus, a small difference between parents and children may have validated the concerns raised in the pilot study and the literature.

Observations about the Data

It is remarkable to note the differences between parent and child perceptions of actual daily stressors. For example, children reported problems with friends and peers with nearly four times the frequency as parents. Children reported the greatest stress about friends, school, siblings, and disappointment, whereas parents perceived disappointment, school, illness, and parental demands to be the greatest child stressors.

Parents perceived their own demands and punishments on children to be stressful nearly two and one-half times more frequently than children reported such stressors. At the same time, parents seemed profoundly less aware of children's concerns with other family members and concerns (as shown by frequencies in the family concerns and family members categories). Parents perceived children to feel the stress of personal responsibility with twice the frequency that children actually reported it. Parents also viewed extracurricular activities to be more frequent stressors than children reported.

Also, although actual frequency in the category of health care visits was relatively low (probably because journal keeping only reflected daily life over a period of 6 weeks), parents were less likely to report the stressor than children, though parents were more likely than children to report a physical symptom as a source of stress. This exemplifies one way in which adults are likely to misinterpret the child's culture. Whereas an adult may see a health care visit as alleviating the stressor of a child's illness, that very event is often a major stressor from the child's point of view. This well-known fact apparently did not affect the parents' personal daily view of their own children. The children's responses appeared to validate the volumes of research on the intense stressors of health care procedures, including hospitalization.

The differences in perceptions between boys and girls are also interesting. Boys identified more situational stressors than did girls, whereas girls reported more stressors related to self and others. Boys listed more stressors related to school, interruptions, and environmental factors. Boys named home chores with nearly four times the frequency of girls, and organizational demands more than twice as often as girls. Girls reported disappointment three times more often than did boys, and personal responsibility two times more often. Among the interpersonal stressors, girls listed friends and siblings, whereas boys listed parental demands and other family members.

CHILDREN'S COPING RESPONSES

Coping data from children's daily journals produced 20 categories. This study validated categories produced earlier by sentence completion (Sorensen, 1990), but also validated the previous observation that frequencies reflecting actual life experience reported in daily journals differ from those expressed in hypothetical sentence completion (Sorensen, 1990, in press-b). Parent journals reflected 13 of the categories that emerged from children's diaries.

The themes of problem-focused (behavioral) and emotion-focused (cognitive) coping responses proposed by Lazarus and Folkman (Folkman, 1979; Lazarus & Folkman, 1984), as well as Murphy's (1974) dichotomy of internal and external coping styles, were found to be inadequate. As categories were inductively identified, the three general domains of cognitive–behavioral, cognitive–intrapsychic, and interpersonal coping efforts emerged as being most congruent with the data from the children. As in the case of stressors, these domains seem to resemble the coping codes of Self, Environment, and Other, used by Wertlieb and associates (1987).

The taxonomy of domains and categories is presented in Table 2,

TABLE 2. Children's Coping Efforts

Domain	Category	Response examples	Total (%)	Girls (%)	Boys (%)	Parents (%)
Cognitive–behavioral	Submission/endurance	"Wait it out," "do [it] anyway," "do what have to"	34.84	26.32	43.35	26.86
	Problem solving	"Solve the problem," "fix [stressor]"	15.86	18.69	13.22	14.92
	Emotional expression	"Cry," "pout," "yell," "scream," "complain"	9.84	12.17	7.51	26.36
	Distraction	"Do something else," "do something fun instead"	5.60	6.58	4.62	2.99
	Behavioral reframing	"Act as if," "pretend to feel," "do my best"	5.46	6.91	4.04	1.49
	Aggression	"Everything went wrong today, so I kicked my sister"	3.88	1.97	5.78	2.99
	Avoidance	"Hide," "run away," "walk away," "go to my room"	2.68	3.62	1.73	4.48
	Rebellion	"Refused to do it," "just didn't do what teacher said"	1.90	0.33	3.47	1.49
	Manipulation/deception	"Beg," "bug," "give excuses," "say my brother did it"	1.85	1.97	1.73	5.97
	Self-effacing	"Suck fingers," "chew nails"	0.79	0.99	0.58	0.00
	Immobilization	"I couldn't move"	0.17	0.00	0.33	0.00
	Subtotal		82.87	79.55	86.36	87.55
Cognitive–intrapsychic	Emotional/sensory	"I feel sad," "shy," "scared," "stupid," "embarrassed"	6.63	9.21	4.04	0.00
	Thought reframing	"Think about [stressor] in a different way"	1.53	1.32	1.73	0.00
	Analyzing/intellectualizing	"Try to figure it out," "think about it"	1.36	0.99	1.73	0.00
	Taking personal responsibility	"It was my fault," "I said I was sorry" "I will do better next time"	1.08	0.99	1.16	0.00
	Emotional/external focus	"Hope for a good grade," "pray for [something]"	0.33	0.66	0.00	1.49
	Subtotal		10.93	13.17	8.66	1.49
Interpersonal	Mother	"Go to Mom," "ask Mom to help"	3.11	3.33	2.89	7.46
	Others	"I asked brother," "went to teacher," "Grandma helped"	1.57	1.97	1.16	1.49
	Friends	"Called my friend," "went to friends," "played with [friend's name]"	1.24	1.32	1.16	0.00
	Mom and Dad	"I asked Mom and Dad"	0.33	0.66	0.00	2.01
	Subtotal		6.25	7.28	5.21	10.96
	TOTAL[a]		100.05	100.00	100.23	100.00

Note. From Sorensen (1990). Copyright 1990 W.B. Saunders Co. Adapted by permission.

[a]Totals not equal to 100.00 due to rounding error.

with specific examples from children's responses, as well as percent frequencies by children and parents. Descriptions of the domains and categories follow.

The Cognitive–Behavioral Domain

This area included categories representing an integration of both cognitive–emotional components and associated behavioral manifestations in coping responses. Though some followers of Lazarus have promoted a separate category of behavioral coping responses, here they were overshadowed by a strong cognitive influence, and so included together.

"Submission/endurance" reflected a resigned emotional acceptance of the stressor situation, whereas responses were described behaviorally, such as "wait it out," or "do what I have to do."

"Problem solving" included approaches where stressors were confronted directly and actively in a behavioral manner. For example, if the source of stress were a lost or broken object, attempts were made to locate or repair the object.

"Emotional expression" included behavioral manifestations of feelings, such as crying or screaming.

"Distraction" behaviors were employed by some to avoid or sublimate the stressor, such as playing with someone else, or doing something other than the activity involving the source of stress.

"Behavioral reframing" reflected activities where the child attempted to change the appraisal or diminish the perception of the stressor, such as by pretending or acting as if the stressor were not a threat.

"Aggression" included physical acts against another, such as hitting or kicking. An interesting example is the boy who wrote, "Everything went wrong today . . . so I kicked my sister."

In "avoidance," the stressor was avoided by hiding, running, or going away to a room, etc.

"Rebellion" reflected a refusal to submit, comply or otherwise "put up with" the reported stressor, or to perform in the face of the perceived demands or injustices of stressor situations.

"Manipulation/deception" activities included purposeful manipulating or deceiving, teasing, bluffing, sneaking, passing blame to a sibling, or purposely denying culpable behavior.

"Self-effacing" behaviors included regressive or comforting personal habits, such as nail-biting or finger sucking.

"Immobilization" reflected responses where the child reported being unable to act or think, as in the stressor situation of feeling unprepared for a school assignment.

The Cognitive–Intrapsychic Domain

This domain embraced those categories reflecting internally focused, emotionally and intellectually centered coping efforts.

"Emotional/sensory" responses were expressions of feelings within, such as fear, sadness, or happiness, with no apparent associated behavioral activities.

"Thought reframing" included intellectual or emotional attempts at thought stopping, changing perceptions, or talking to self to reframe perceptions.

"Analyzing/intellectualizing" coping efforts were cognitive problem-focused attempts at problem solving, without apparent behavioral outcomes. Such responses included thinking, figuring out, or planning responses to stressors.

"Taking personal responsibility" embraced cognitive–behavioral self-focusing activities, such as self-blame, apologizing, or actions to personally improve a situation.

"Emotional/external focus" included emotional responses directed outside of self, rather than centered on feelings within. Externally focused responses included worrying *about* something, or praying or wishing *for* something, though responses were not acted upon behaviorally.

The Interpersonal Coping Domain

These categories included coping efforts where social support was the significant factor. Support was sought specifically from those in the following categories: "Mother"; "others," including siblings, teachers, and grandparents; "friends"; and "Mom and Dad," who appeared to be perceived as a unit.

It is interesting to note that whereas several children reported seeking help specifically from the mother as a coping strategy and a few wrote in "Mom and Dad" as a unit, none reported going specifically to the father for social support as a coping response.

Observations about the Data

The most common response reported by boys, girls, and parents to actual daily stressors was submission or endurance, reflecting a general perception of either (1) children's lack of control over most daily phenomena, or (2) the reality that most daily stress phenomena simply must be accepted. Boys reported significantly more submission/ endurance than girls or parents, with 43% of all boys' coping responses falling into that category. Parents and children also generally agreed, according to the frequency of their reports, that after submission/ endurance the two most common coping responses were problem solving and emotional expression.

Parent–child differences in reporting coping efforts were interesting. Parents listed only one of the five categories reported by children among the cognitive–intrapsychic, or emotion-focused, coping responses. In other words, parents simply failed to notice the children's inner responses of emotional feeling, thinking, reframing, or assuming a sense of responsibility. Parents were more likely to notice the children's manipulation/deception than children reported, and also more likely than the children to report social support seeking (especially from mothers). However, parents did not notice the importance of children's friends in coping.

It is significant that boys were most likely to record submission/ endurance, whereas girls recorded more problem-solving coping efforts. However, in the cognitive–intrapsychic domain, boys recorded more analyzing/intellectualizing and taking personal responsibility. Girls were about twice as likely as boys to report emotional/sensory and emotional expression. Boys reported rebellion and physical aggression as stress responses, whereas girls were more likely to use avoidance, distraction, and behavioral reframing.

CHILDREN'S COPING RESOURCES/UPLIFTS

Coping resources were identified as "buffers" (Sorensen, 1991) or those situations, people, events, or activities listed in the daily journals as the "best part of the day." They were described by the family as those factors that helped most in dealing with the life experiences of the day, and were interpreted as mediating variables that reduced the effects of stressors or enhanced coping. Data revealed 16 categories in children's reports of coping resources, emerging from the three major domains of social–physical activities, personal satisfaction/comfort, and social support. Parent responses fell into only 13 of those categories, and produced no additional ones. The taxonomy of domains and categories, refined from those previously derived (Sorensen, 1991) is presented in Table 3. Descriptions of the categories follow.

TABLE 3. Children's Coping Resources/Uplifts

Domain	Category	Children (%)	Girls (%)	Boys (%)	Parents (%)
Social-physical	Organized activity	17.38	15.43	19.33	10.99
activities	School subjects	16.05	18.49	13.60	7.69
	Sports	6.17	0.64	11.69	2.20
	Unexpected activity	2.84	2.57	3.10	0.00
	Subtotal	42.44	37.13	47.72	20.88
Personal	Free play	9.07	6.43	11.70	14.29
satisfaction/	Feeling of				
comfort	accomplishment	8.10	11.41	4.78	13.19
	Physical comfort	6.68	6.43	6.92	14.29
	Release from				
	responsibilities	6.41	7.56	5.25	5.49
	Being at home	4.32	3.86	4.78	1.10
	Getting something				
	new	1.96	2.73	1.19	3.30
	Weather	0.32	0.16	0.48	5.49
	Subtotal	36.86	38.58	35.10	57.15
Social support	Friends	12.80	13.67	11.93	15.39
	Relatives	4.93	6.27	3.58	5.49
	Mother	1.20	1.45	0.95	0.00
	Father	0.97	1.45	0.48	0.00
	School teacher	0.85	1.45	0.24	1.10
	Subtotal	20.75	24.29	17.18	21.98
	TOTAL[a]	100.05	100.00	100.00	100.01

[a]All totals not equal to 100.00 due to rounding error.

Social-Physical Activities

This area included group activities, generally where both physical activity and peer relations were involved.

"Organized activity" was the category reported with the greatest frequency. Included were such activities as school or church social gatherings, scouting activities, parties, concerts, and going out to eat, in which the child was involved in a family or peer group.

"School subjects" or events included physical education (listed with the greatest frequency), recess, art, music, science, and mathematics.

"Sports," such as soccer, football, and baseball (both formally and informally organized), were mentioned more frequently by boys than girls.

"Unexpected activities" included both informal activities or surprise events, in which the child had not expected to participate, or unexpected attention from an adult, such as a teacher. The element of pleasant surprise seemed to be the essential buffer. Diary examples included "I got to ride on a truck" or "today I was chosen to ring the bell."

Personal Satisfaction/Comfort

Resources or uplifts under the domain of personal satisfaction/comfort seemed to reflect emotionally and intellectually satisfying situations, and conditions of personal physical comfort. Several of the responses implied uplifts in a sense of control or self-esteem.

"Free play" included individual, self-motivated, and self-initiated projects, where the child was allowed freedom of choice in the selection of activities. Examples included starting a club and "getting to play whatever I wanted."

"Feelings of accomplishment," or sense of competence, were identified usually following task completion or positive performance. Journal examples were "I got the job done, made a home run, had a good piano lesson, homework was done on time, I scored in soccer." It should be noted that in the children's diaries these responses were reported from the internal perspective of the child, rather than from adult feedback. Positive feedback from others falls under the domain of social support.

"Physical comfort" included simple daily pleasures, such as bathing, sleep, and favorite foods. Foods listed by children were burritos, doughnuts, ice cream, candy, cookies, pizza, and caramel apples.

"Release from responsibilities," such as chores, demands, or routines, was usually granted by either circumstance or by authority figures, and was perceived as a resource. Such diary entries stated, "no homework, didn't owe lunch money, school was out early, no science today."

"Being at home" was a category in which children recorded pleasure at being with parents, siblings, and pets.

"Getting something new," either planned or as a surprise, was a perceived uplift. Items listed included a lamp, new bed, eyeglasses, book, and stickers.

"Weather" conditions included reports of a sunny day or new snow.

Social Support

As mentioned earlier, seeking social support was listed as a coping strategy. However, the availability of social support, even when not actively sought, was also listed as a stress mediator. Sources of social support included the following:

"Friends" — playing, talking, calling, and planning with peers
"Relatives" — grandparents, cousins, aunts, and uncles
"Mother" and "father" — for example, "A good thing about today was that Mom was home."
"Teacher" — personal attention from a school teacher

Observations about the Data

The area of coping resources/uplifts proved to be the most intriguing element in the exploration. Both parents and children recorded responses in this area with the greatest frequency. The area began with the idea of "resources," and evolved, based on journal responses, toward the idea of "uplifts." The importance of the mediating variables listed in this area is underscored by the frequency with which they were identified and expressed in the family diaries.

The themes in coping resources/uplifts are closely related to coping strategies outlined by other scholars. Resources of intrapsychic comfort, found in the domain of personal satisfaction/comfort, parallel the intrapsychic or cognitive coping themes identified by Lazarus and Folkman (1984), Caty and associates (1984), Sorensen (1991), and Walker (1988). The social–physical activities and physical comfort buffers relate to some of the behavioral coping responses discussed by the same authors.

In addition, the importance of social support was also validated in this study. However, the possibility emerged of a delineation between social support that is sought (as shown in Table 2) and social support that is recognized as available and helpful (as shown in Table 3).

Children reported organized activities as the most common daily personal resource. Although parents listed organized activities with considerable frequency, they listed friends as the most frequent resource for children. Parents were more likely to report free play, feelings of accomplishment, and physical comfort than children. It is interesting to note that parents failed to notice surprise activities as a daily resource for children. Parents also did not note themselves as sources of social support.

There are some interesting gender differences that provide important clues to those attempting to mediate stress in children. In specific categories, girls reported school subjects, feelings of accomplishment, release from responsibilities, and getting something new more often than boys. Boys listed organized activities, sports, free play, and weather conditions most often. Thus, girls were generally more likely to report cognitive intrapsychic or social support resources, whereas boys were more likely to list physical activities and environmental factors.

When listing a school subject, either as a source of stress or as an uplift for the day, both boys and girls mentioned physical education most often. Usually when adults were asked to name the school subject causing the greatest stress to children, they chose mathematics, science, or spelling. When asked to name the school subject that offers the greatest uplift to children, frequent responses from adults were art, music, or recess.

Perhaps only by remembering childhood can adults perceive the stress of physical activities for children. Not being chosen for a team or missing the ball probably constitute greater stressors for children than simply struggling with a problem in mathematics. Furthermore, it seems that the uplift of succeeding in a physical education class far outweighs the adult-perceived pleasure of singing a song in music class.

NOTES ON THE TAXONOMIES

These beginning taxonomies identify and organize the rich data on stress–coping phenomena in children. In the areas of stressors, coping responses, and resources/uplifts, three major themes emerged—external, internal, and social orientations. Table 4 outlines the taxonomies according to the following themes:

1. External themes of situational stressors, visible cognitive–behavioral coping efforts, and social–physical uplifts
2. Internal themes of self-focused stressors, cognitive–intrapsychic emotion-focused coping responses, and personal satisfaction/comfort uplifts
3. Social themes of others-focused stressors, interpersonal coping responses, and social support resources

Table 5 documents the subtotal frequencies among children and parents, represented as percentages, among the major domains of the taxonomies. Although Table 5 reflects no clear-cut patterns in relationships among the domains, we gain some information from the frequency comparisons. First, although parents' reports on external coping responses came close to the frequency of children's reports, the parents did not adequately recognize the cognitive–intrapsychic coping responses among children. This may indicate that adults tend to view

TABLE 4. Outline of Stress-Coping Taxonomies

Themes	Stressors	Coping responses	Resources/uplifts
External	Situations School Home chores Interruption Organizational demands Environmental discomfort Health care visits	Cognitive- behavioral Submission/ endurance Problem solving Emotional expression Distraction Behavioral reframing Aggression Avoidance Rebellion Manipulation/ deception Self-effacing Immobilization	Social–physical activities Organized activity School subjects Sports Unexpected activity
Internal	Self Disappointment Physical symptoms Cognitive- emotional discomforts Personal responsibility	Cognitive- intrapsychic Emotional/ sensory Thought reframing Analyzing/ intellectualizing Taking personal responsibility Emotional/ external focus	Personal satisfaction/ comfort Free play Feeling of accomplishment Physical comfort Release from responsibilities Being at home Getting something new Weather
Social	Others Friends Siblings Parental demands Family concerns School teacher Family members	Interpersonal Mother Others Friends Mom and Dad	Social support Friends Relatives Mother Father School teacher

responses to stress in terms of visible behavioral management, whereas children are more likely to accept a cognitive or emotional responses as a legitimate way of dealing with stress.

A second interesting observation is that parents are able to approximate the frequency of children's reports of social support as coping responses and coping resources, but not in the identification of other people as perceived sources of stress to children.

TABLE 5. Responses by Percentage among General Taxonomy Themes

Themes	Stressors		Coping responses		Resources/Uplifts	
	Children	Parents	Children	Parents	Children	Parents
External	Situations		Cognitive–behavioral		Social–physical activities	
	34.39	41.99	75.52	87.55	43.73	20.88
Internal	Self		Cognitive–intrapsychic		Personal satisfaction/comfort	
	30.23	42.35	14.84	1.49	35.84	57.15
Social	Others		Interpersonal		Social support	
	35.38	15.66	9.64	10.96	20.25	21.98

Tables 6, 7, and 8 represent a collapsing of children's and parents' reports of external, internal, and social (1) stressors with coping responses and (2) stressors with coping resources, and (3) resources with coping. This attempt at cross-tabulation was done by calculating the means between parents and children and among the domains of all areas, then redistributing the combined means so that each entire table adds to 100%. This allows a simplified descriptive view of the possible relationships among the themes of stressors, coping responses, and resources.

TABLE 6. Stressors Related to Coping by Theme

		Coping		
		Internal	External	Social
Stressors				
Internal		7.43	19.68	7.79
External		7.75	20.00	7.79
Social		5.64	17.89	5.99
TOTAL	99.96[a]			

[a]Total does not add to 100.00 due to rounding error.

TABLE 7. Stressors Related to Resources by Theme

		Resources		
		Internal	External	Social
Stressors				
Internal		13.80	11.44	9.57
External		14.12	11.76	9.89
Social		12.01	9.65	7.78
TOTAL	100.02[a]			

[a]Total does not add to 100.00 due to rounding error.

TABLE 8. Resources Related to Coping by Theme

| | | Coping | |
	Internal	External	Social
Resources			
Internal	9.11	21.35	9.47
External	6.75	18.98	7.10
Social	4.88	17.12	5.24
TOTAL 100.00			

Table 6 indicates that external coping responses are the most frequently employed with all the themes among stressors. However, Table 7 shows that all areas of stressors are most frequently associated with internal types of resources or uplifts. The greatest frequencies were reported in the areas of internal resources and external coping (21.35 — see Table 8) and external coping with external stressors (20.00 — see Table 6). It is not clear what this may mean, except perhaps that external sources of stress and coping are more visible and easily reported by parents and children.

The least frequent associations were social resources with internal coping responses (4.88 — see Table 8), social resources with social coping efforts (5.24 — see Table 8), social stressors with social coping efforts (5.99 — see Table 6), and social stressors with internal coping efforts (5.64 — see Table 6). These seem to indicate that children and parents are likely to identify social support with least frequency as a resource or means of coping, and that both adults and children report visible environmental conditions and behavioral responses more than internal cognitive-emotional events.

Again, it must be noted that caution must be exercised in such generalizations from quantifications in this study. Frequencies only indicate the incidence of reports of descriptive daily experiences.

An Overview of the Taxonomies

The themes and categories derived from this exploration exhibited some differences and similarities with other inductive works. Lewis et al. (1984) did not identify general domains for stressors, but developed a list of stressors by psychometric methods. Many items in their list (examples include problems with parents, homework, being late, not good at sports, etc.) were also reported by the children in this study.

Band and Weisz (1988) listed stressor themes similar to those included in my taxonomy. Among those are medical procedures, peer difficulties, and school problems. Dickey and Henderson (1989) noted school work, peer relationships, teacher relationships, family events, personal injury, loss of personal comfort, and discipline, all of which are similar to categories revealed in this investigation.

Stressor areas identified in the literature that were not reported by the children in this project include parental marital difficulties, change of residence, and parental illness. This may be because the diaries documented only a 6-week period.

In the area of coping, the concept of submission/endurance is found as endurance (Dise-Lewis, 1988), relinquishment (Band & Weisz, 1988), and acceptance (Dickey & Henderson, 1989). Problem solving has been called direct problem solving and direct action (Band & Weisz, 1988; Dickey & Henderson, 1989). Emotional expression, distraction, reframing, aggression, and seeking social support have been observed by the same authors cited here, as well as Walker (1988) and Ryan (1989).

Similarities and discrepancies among the results of this study and others need to be examined more closely for logical consistency, and perhaps integrated and tested. The internal and external, cognitive and behavioral foci of coping responses resembled Murphy's (1974) observations of coping styles as (1) the capacity to deal with the environment, and (2) the capacity to maintain internal equilibrium.

Coping categories identified here resembled those developed by Caty and associates (1984) — action/inaction (which can be construed as behavioral) and intrapsychic (which coincides with cognitive). Such similarities reflect consistency within the general cognitive–transactional model for stress–coping research.

This examination identified some of the same coping categories as Dise-Lewis (1984) and Ryan (1989), plus many more. In view of these findings the attempts of those authors at instrument development may be premature.

Although other taxonomies of stressors and coping efforts exist in the literature, as discussed, there is no list of coping resources from the viewpoint of the subjects as derived here. The concept of resources as presented here needs to be validated further.

This exploration also offered information beyond the simple narrative description and categorization provided by previous qualitative studies. The frequency tables allowed a view of the proportions of responses in various categories and the numerical relationship among variables. Hopefully, this kind of data presentation and interpretation can provide a foundation for hypothesis construction and testing, but it needs replication and refinement. Data obtained in this way could be used for instrument development and standardization.

Individual appraisal significantly influenced analysis and taxonomy development. The types of stressor appraisals listed by Folkman and Lazarus (1984) — harm-loss, threat, and challenge, as well as simple annoyance — were evident across all categories. Indeed, as proposed by Lazarus, appraisal seemed to be the chief determining variable in responding to a given stressor.

Differences in appraisal are seen in the following examples from the diaries.

To the situation, "Mom and Dad are not home," responses indicating positive appraisal or challenge included:

"I can play."
"I can watch what I want on television."
"They are probably at the mall."
"That's good."

Appraisals of threat included:

"I think about them."
"I should lock the door."
"I worry."
"I think about scary things."

Harm-loss responses included the following:

"I hope they are not dead."
"I think they are never coming back."
"They are having fun and I am not."

Differences in appraisal were also seen in feelings expressed about the first day of school: weird, worried, funny, terrible, shy, embarrassed, scared, left out, fine, good, happy, excited.

To the stressor of breaking something, children responded with emotional responses ("get chills . . . get upset . . . feel sad . . . panic . . . cry"), behavioral responses indicating an appraisal of threat ("get in trouble . . . hide . . . run away"), behavioral responses showing an appraisal of challenge ("get a new one . . . try to fix it"), and interpersonal responses ("tell someone . . . tell Mom . . . tell the owner").

PARENTAL PERCEPTIONS OF CHILD STRESS EXPERIENCES: ANOTHER VIEW OF THE DATA

We must develop theory that reflects either (1) the uniqueness of the childhood experience and/or (2) the distinctive position, perspective, and contribution of the child in the family. A critical step is to determine how adults' perceptions of stress and coping in specific situations resemble or differ from the perceptions of the children themselves. Parents' ability to accurately perceive the stress experiences of their own children plays an important role in the capacity of parents to respond appropriately to the needs of their children. Furthermore, we cannot claim to understand the family without examining the views of both the parents and children.

Knutson (1991), performing a secondary analysis on data from this study, examined the ability of parents to adopt the perspective of their own children in specific stress experiences. As discussed in Chapter 3, concepts similar to "perspective taking" are found in literature about communication, child development, problem solving, management, and practitioner–patient relationships. These concepts include empathy or role taking. The concept of "maternal thinking" is found in feminist literature (Ruddick, 1982). However, the concept of parent-to-child perspective taking seems to be distinct from those listed. Loosely defined, it is the ability to take another person's point of view, across developmental roles, across caretaker–dependent roles, and across familial patterns and expectations.

Thus Knutson (1991) disregarded domains and taxonomies, and instead examined patterns of parent–child perspective taking. She approached the data asking the question, "To what degree did the parent journals show agreement with or similarity to child journals in describing daily stress–coping experiences?" Knutson attempted to view stress–coping phenomena as a more holistic stress–coping *experience* and tried to ascertain the degree of agreement among family members on given days and over time.

Knutson also assigned parental scores based on the degree of agreement with children's reports, and then described patterns and themes that emerged from parents who (1) scored high in agreement or similarity, and who (2) scored low in agreement or similarity. The child's diary entries were thus used as the standard for the validity of the stress-experience report.

Knutson examined 1,028 same-day child–parent journal pairs from 43 children of the entire original data set. Of the parental journal entries, 60 (5.84%) were from fathers, and all others were from mothers. She found that parent–child agreement or similarity occurred in no more than 48.19% of all parent–child diaries. Knutson further attempted to correlate agreement/similarity in the areas of stressors, coping responses, and uplifts, finding coping and uplifts to be the least correlated ($r = .36-.49$). Ironically, coping and uplifts have appeared to be most related theoretically.

Different themes emerged between parents with low agreement scores and those with high agreement. Among parents with low agreement, Knutson identified the three major patterns: "Projection," "Justification," and "Too Busy."

The pattern of Projection involves situations in which parents presume elements of their own experience to be the experience of their child. Knutson describes an example:

> The younger sister threw the older sister's new shoes away. . . . On that day, the older sister and the mother recorded the incident as "the thing that upset the child most that day." The younger sister reported a different stress entirely, and seemed to be less affected. The following day, neither of the girls made reference to the [shoe] incident, but the mother still reported it as both girls "upset" for the day. The parent wrote . . . "She'd better learn from it" in one journal. In the other journal the mother responded, "still mad about yesterday and the shoes," adding that what the child "did about it" was "I hope learned from it!" It seems that it was the mother who was still upset, not the children. (p. 43)

The pattern of Justification represents situations in which parents used their own journals as a vehicle to rationalize, justify, or exonerate parental behavior that may have influenced the child's journal. Knutson pointed out that although events described may have been similar, agreement on the perception of the stress–coping experience was quite different. The following excerpt illustrates this idea (Knutson, 1991):

> The first example of this kind of response is a parent who indicated that the child's stress for that day was "not being allowed to wear this *outrageous* outfit in public," and the child's coping as "decided she *could live* only wearing it for play." Note the tone of justification and minimization in the mother's responses. The child, on the other hand, reports, "My mom would not let me wear the clothes I wanted." (p. 44)

Too Busy emerged as a theme among low-scoring families. In such parental journals, there was no apparent attempt to rationalize or justify. Parents showed no signs of frustration, but simply seemed too busy, distracted, or inattentive to connect with the child's perception. Knutson related a classic illustration of this pattern — on the day when the child reported the stressor of the day to be "everything," the parent wrote, "none that I know of" (p. 45).

Patterns among parents scoring high in agreement with the child's perception of stress experiences included (1) high incidence and agreement on "the no stressor response," (2) "child as informant," and (3) score consistency.

Knutson noticed that among those children who reported "no stressor," or "nothing" in response to the questions of the semistructured journals, there were a number whose parents showed a high incidence of agreement for the same days. She further noticed that parent–child pairs who reported consistent agreement on no stress also consistently agreed on uplifts. There seemed to be some clinical significance to the pattern of (1) the parent–child agreement, (2) the apparent relative "absence" of stress, and (3) high agreement in reports of uplifts in such families.

The "Child as Informant" pattern described situations where there was high agreement between parent and child journals, but on issues and topics to which parents could not have had direct access. Examples include situations in school, with friends, or children's private experiences. Knutson reports (1991), "Some parents accurately matched their child's uplift responses day after day, reporting things such as specific parts of the school day, conversations with friends, and specifics about the child's emotions relative to a particular experience" (p. 47). In such cases, it was apparent that parents had sought or been given an inside view into the child's perspective. Knutson assumed that the child had served as an informant, "letting parents in" to their world view, though particularly attentive parents might have gained information from other sources.

The third theme emerging from high-scoring parents was that of score consistency between agreement and similarity on Knutson's scales. That is, when high-scoring parents described their child's stress experience, they seemed able to see it from the child's viewpoint, agreeing in detail. When journals of high-agreement parents did not agree with the child's view, they tended to miss the target entirely, describing a totally different experience. In other words, high-scoring parents did not describe similar situations from a different point of view. They either were "right on" to the child's view, or missed it.

Knutson's analysis of parents' abilities to take the perspective of the child raises several issues. First, with such an apparent range of parental abilities to reflect the child's worldview, familiar questions about methods that measure "family" perceptions again emerge. If the child's perspective is to be included in family observations, methods must move beyond adult-report paper–pencil tests. Second, one theme underlying Knutson's interpretations seems to be family type or style, validating the importance of such variables in the study of family stress–coping phenomena. Finally, individual differences continue to appear as important variables in family study.

SUMMARY AND CONCLUSIONS

This chapter has presented the results of a study of 42 well, school-age children and their parents. From the analysis of daily semistructured journals, the qualitative, descriptive design produced the beginning of taxonomies of children's daily stressors—which resemble hassles; coping responses—cognitive-emotional, behavioral, and social; and personal coping resources, or uplifts. Further, the analysis of daily child–parent journals revealed several themes related to the ability of parents to assume the perspective of the child.

The semistructured daily journals proved to be an efficient, effective method for collecting subjective data from several family members over time. Journals provided a means, which was neither intrusive nor artificial, to observe realities from several perspectives. The diaries allowed the children to respond authentically without attempting to predict investigator expectations or relying on hypothetical situations, as might occur in an isolated interview situation. Compliance in journal keeping was highest in the children, followed by the mothers, with few fathers participating.

The limitations of the method included the inability of the investigator to get information in addition to diary entries. For example, I was unable to probe into the situation of the boy who wrote, "Everything went wrong today, so I kicked my sister." Whether the entry indicated a subtle, serious problem in family relationships, an aggressive personality, or even an interesting sense of humor could not be ascertained.

The data base needs to be increased for accurate instrument development and theory refinement. Categories found here were deliberately left broad and varied. Concept definition is still developing and evidence of that challenge is found in the report. There remains considerable investigator ambivalence about methods of data analysis. When should one crunch the numbers in search for statistical significance and when should one simply allow the rich meaning to emerge from the narrative?

Further study can identify the relationships among variables and among the reported data from various family members. Neither the severity of the stressors nor the effectiveness of particular coping responses was determined, and these need scholarly attention before any valid prescriptions for prevention or intervention can be developed.

However, given an effective vehicle, it is evident from this exploration that school-age children can articulate private perceptions, that data can be drawn from more than one family member, and that subjective reports from well people can offer valuable information.

Learning from Children's Art

A glimpse into the subjective world view of schoolage children is available through their nonverbal, symbolic expressions in art. Ironically, although the social sciences have eagerly embraced conceptual symbols in family theory and research, visual symbols have received less attention. Recently, however, in the disciplines of child development, psychology, and education, a recognition of children's art as a significant part of childhood language has emerged. Art therapy has also become a recognized discipline in its own right (Rubin, 1984). The value of broadening multidisciplinary approaches to family studies (particularly when the focus is on children) is further underscored.

The use of an aesthetic, intuitive mode, such as art, in assessment or therapy lies on the opposite end of the continuum from more readily quantifiable, positivistic methods. But, in the study of children, the importance of art as symbolic language cannot be denied (DiLeo, 1970, 1983). Lowenfeld and Brittain (1975) observed that a child's art is an extension and reflection of his or her reality. Art images may offer clues to the child's perception of self, as well as areas of stress, conflict, or need.

Speaking of children's art from an aesthetic perspective, Rafael Goldin, director of the International Museum of Children's Art in Oslo, Norway asserted:

> To respect children is very important. This, people don't understand. People [formerly] didn't look at the creations of childhood. It was a blank space on the map. Children may not be able to speak to us in our language. But *their* language is wonderful. What they express is a stage in our lives that we can't return to, and at the very moment they experience it. These are the originals. (Shenker, 1990, p. 148)

Art has particular advantages in a descriptive study of children, where meaning is sought. It offers a unique permanence of expression that is not distorted by memory, and may also provide a record of processes over time. To the children, it is a helpful supplement to linear communication of verbalization by providing a spatial matrix for communication (Wadeson, 1980).

Children's art has been used in assessment, diagnosis, and therapy as a means to help children gain self-awareness and nurture creative processes (Rubin, 1984; Wadeson, 1980; Wilson & Ratekin, 1990), and simply for its aesthetic, intuitive information about children.

The use of such a subjective, even intuitive, measure as art seemed to lose favor with the surge of positivistic approaches in the social sciences a few decades ago. However, new activity in qualitative methods has created a resurgence of interest in art analysis and therapy. Much of the recent work in children's art assessment has been done in England and Europe (see examples: Case & Dalley, 1990; Dalley et al., 1987; Delgorgue & Engelhart, 1984; Lucio del Raggi & Huazo, 1984; Miljkovitch, 1984–1985; Tholome, 1984–1985).

ART IN PROJECTIVE ASSESSMENT TECHNIQUES

The history of drawing as an assessment tool parallels the history of other pediatric projective techniques including story telling, the Rorschach inkblot technique, sentence completion tests, and particular drawing tasks (Chandler, & Johnson, 1991; Fine, 1978; Johnson, 1990; Krahn, 1985).

Art assessment has been formalized by the development of several objective instruments for analyzing children's art according to projective theory. Many of these include analysis and numerical scoring systems for particular drawing tasks whose content generally includes human figures, houses, or trees (Brumback, 1977; Hartman, 1972; Kuhlman & Bieliauskas, 1976; Riordan & Verdel, 1991). Children's drawings of the human figure have been analyzed for reflections of gender perception (Zucker, Finegan, Doering, & Bradley, 1983), self-esteem (Coopersmith, Sakai, Beardslee, & Coopersmith, 1976; Prytula & Thompson, 1973), and body image (Nathan, 1973).

Koppitz (1983) outlined the value of children's drawings as a projective assessment technique in a number of areas. Human figure drawings can reflect personality characteristics, and family drawings offer insights into children's attitudes toward parents, siblings, and perceptions of their place in their own families. School drawings give clues to attitudes toward teachers, peers, and school. Thus, art offers a general reflection of social and cultural values and attitudes.

Much of the literature on projective drawings among children examines disturbed, maladjusted, or ill children, who may have special needs complicated by diminished expressive abilities (Brandell, 1986; Howe, Burgess, & McCormack, 1987; Miljkovitch & Irvine, 1982). For example, there has been considerable attention to the drawings of children who are victims of abuse (Malchiodi, 1990; Manning, 1987; Schornstein & Derr, 1978), particularly sexual abuse (Briggs & Lehmann, 1989; Cohen & Phelps, 1985; Riordan & Verdel, 1991).

Drawings have also been used in family assessment (Smith, 1985; Tholome, 1984–1985) to evaluate individual functioning within the context of the family. Straus (1964) used projective techniques with families in research, but mostly in clinical diagnosis. Straus called such tests "disguised-voluntary measures" (p. 374); the informant is asked to respond to unstructured pictures, such as ink blots, cartoons, and other types of drawings. Similar projective techniques used to explore relationships in family assessment may include play situations, interplay with three-dimensional shapes, and clay sculpting. Such use of art in individual and family diagnosis has a long history of validation and refinement.

Recently, the kinetic family drawing technique has probably drawn the most attention as a projective assessment tool (Jones, 1985; Mostkoff & Lazarus, 1983; Stawar & Stawar, 1987). Knoff and Prout (1985) reviewed studies using such techniques. Art therapy has also been used in the family group setting for creative function, to heighten or lower affective states, to influence freedom of self-expression, to circumvent defenses, and to facilitate family interactions, cooperation, attitudes of openness, and insights (Landgarten, 1987).

USE OF SPONTANEOUS DRAWINGS

Although most of the studies cited here have used projective methods, there is an increasing interest in children's spontaneous art work. Indeed, Hargreaves (1978) questioned the attempted objectivity of traditional projective approaches, proposing instead a process orientation to children's self-initiated art work. Furth (1988) and Baker (1991) have studied impromptu drawings and paintings of terminally ill, hospitalized, and well children. McNiff (1982) examined sex differences in children's spontaneous drawings, noting interesting differences in subject matter and style between boys and girls, without finding the expected stereotypical images of sex roles. Hurwitz (1980) noted cultural differences in children's art.

Assessment versus Therapy

The lines between assessment, diagnosis, and therapy are thin and ill-defined. Kramer (1971) emphasized the integrative and healing processes of the creative process itself, which does not require verbal reflection and works especially well with children. The assessment process can become effective therapy, as children are able to release tension through lines, colors, and forms (Malchiodi, 1990; Rubin, 1984; Shrewsbury, 1982; Steinhardt, 1989).

Art has provided a means of self-expression to people suffering terminal illness (Kiepenheuer, 1980; Siegel, 1986; Tate, 1989). Art assessment and therapy have been used effectively with terminally ill and bereaved children (Baker, 1991; Bluestein, 1978; Furth, 1988; Segal, 1984). Indeed, well-known works in art analysis have been done with the critically ill (Bach, 1966, 1975; Kubler-Ross, 1981). Messages from the art of distressed children can be poignant and powerful.

Validity and Ethical Concerns

Validity and the ethical implications of children's art analysis are important issues. There is some controversy among professionals about the appropriate use of children's drawings. There are concerns about bias in interpretation and the fallibility of subjective human judgment in analysis (Martin, 1983; Paterson & Janzen, 1984). Blomeyer (1978) documented that the results of children's art analysis are unconsciously determined to some degree by the interviewer. A study of 1,000 drawings produced 300 interviews with children by 20 professional interviewers, and the findings indicated that children interviewed by the same person produced drawings similar in handwriting and content, even without explicit requests for content. Krahn (1985) also noted that the usefulness of projective art techniques is dependent on the individual skill and interpretation of the clinician. However, noting the reliability of some criteria for art analysis, Levenberg (1975), in a study of kinetic family drawings of 36 normal and disturbed children, found no difference in the overall diagnostic accuracy or the degree of confidence among doctorally prepared clinicians, predoctoral interns, and hospital secretaries.

Riordan and Verdel (1991) proposed the integration of art and children's verbal descriptions, and noted that professionals need to thoroughly understand the normal development of children's artistic progression. Falk (1981) further asserted that art analysis ought to be accepted and documented as an intuitive means of understanding children. In a critical analysis of traditional projective techniques with accompanying attempts at objective scoring criteria, Falk noted that the traditional use of art analysis may contradict the original theory and intended application of projective techniques, and promote the inappropriate use of psychodiagnostic labels. Thus, the analysis of spontaneous art work, in contrast to structured projected techniques, is on the rise.

Criteria for the Analysis of Symbols

Art therapists and others have noticed particular symbols to be important in children's drawings. Siegel (1986) noted

> two important symbols—the rainbow and the butterfly. In dreams, mythology, and art, the rainbow is a symbol of hope and a manifestation of our entire emotional spectrum and life. The butterfly is a universal symbol of metamorphosis. . . . Children in a Nazi concentration camp scratched butterflies on the walls of their cells. (p. 118)

Baker (1991) also noted the transformation symbol of the butterfly.

Bach (1966) and Kubler-Ross (1981) studied symbols created by dying children who were allowed a free choice of form, color, and design. Baker (1991) reported symbols of death awareness such as consistent color frequency (black in monsters, spiders, and snakes, and red in blood), the setting sun, drawn in the upper left corner, and the "soul window" of a house. Many terminally ill children who drew houses showed evidence of their own disease in their house figure. Other symbols, such as numbers of objects, missing body parts, barriers, and so forth, have been noted among children with emotional trauma (Furth, 1988; Malchiodi, 1990).

CHILDREN'S ART IN THIS STUDY

The analysis of children's art in this study was not based on a standardized objective or numerical scoring system, as are some projective methods. Criteria for interpretation were few, beyond those generally accepted in the literature (Bach, 1975; Baker, 1991; Furth, 1988; Rubin, 1984). It should be noted that most guidelines for the analysis of children's art emerge from studies of children who have experienced extreme trauma, such as death, terminal illness, or abuse. The art represented in this study is from children who were assumed to be physically and emotionally healthy. Thus, similarities in symbolism and intensity may not be evident between children in this study and children reported in other works.

Drawings were examined for the general tone and feeling of the art, especially in relation to the associated written diary entry. General content was explored whether it included apparently positive or negative images. The art was explored for unusual items, items out of place, barriers (such as trees, people, walls, lines, etc.), proportion and emphasis of particular objects, or repeated objects. Relative size, detail, and position of human figures, especially if they seemed to depict the child artist, were considered important. Because all children had access to twelve colors, the use of color was especially important in analysis.

Further, it must be acknowledged that I did not have the benefit of verbal dialogue with children about their drawings, relying only on their diary entries. Generally, this would be considered a weakness in interpretation. Indeed, some have viewed the child–researcher interaction and child's explanation of drawings as essential (Deatrick & Faux, 1991; Furth, 1988). On the other hand, the children were not influenced by the investigator's presence while the drawings were produced. Although some nuances may have been missed because of the lack of verbal dialogue, the art here, accompanied by journal entries, seems to speak for itself.

The drawings from the children of this study offered delightful glimpses into the day-to-day world of the child and the family. However, drawings are presented and discussed only to offer insights; diagnosis cannot be made on the basis of a few drawings. The purpose of the artwork in this study was not diagnosis, but enrichment, as children's art can offer an important avenue for nonverbal communication. The drawings are offered only to enhance the general phenomenological picture of coping in children and families. Therefore, although art is a powerful medium, one must not attach too much meaning to the drawings presented.

Examples provided reflect the broad range of drawings that children produced from day to day, and the changes in tone and content therein.

Each child in the study was given a set of 12 colored markers for daily drawings, thus providing the same medium and color choices to all children. Landgarten (1987) asserted that markers and pencils provide children with a high degree of control in art expression, as opposed to the lesser control of water colors or even crayons.

The total number of drawings was 616 (indicating that 49.8% of diary entries included a drawing). Boys provided 267 drawings, or an average of 15.7% per child, and girls provided 349 drawings, with a mean of 14.0% per girl. Following is a discussion of a handful of typical drawings. The nine drawings selected for presentation here reflect themes typical of all the children. Although the richness of color is sacrificed to the black-and-white format, these nine drawings were also selected because they send their message powerfully even without original color.

In Figure 1, we see a profusion of lines flowing from the mouth of a girl, evidently confronting a boy. This is the work of an 11-year-old girl whose diary entry for the day was, "Tyler told my secret. I told him off!" The quickly drawn, black, primitive human figures present a picture of frustration. However, both people have bright yellow hair and blue eyes. Note that in the drawing the girl is not backing away from Tyler, but she, a bit larger than her foe, is apparently confidently confronting the source of her stress at that moment. The child expresses some competence and autonomy in her written diary entry and in other clues in the drawing.

The perception of control in a child's life was a frequent theme in the drawings. Figure 2 portrays a 9-year-old girl's perception of control, with a corresponding diary entry: "My dad and mom did not let me play today." A simple stop sign, with letters filled in in red, stands on an infinite black line, offering insight into her sense of helplessness in this particular situation.

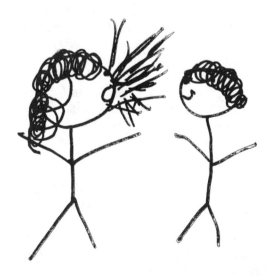

FIGURE 1. "Tyler told my secret. I told him off!"

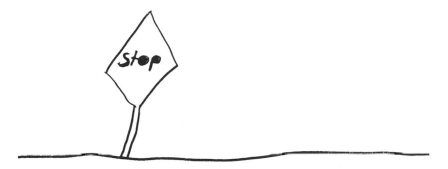

FIGURE 2. "My dad and mom did not let me play today."

Similarly, in Figure 3 an 8-year-old boy depicts a moment of powerlessness. His image, nearly hidden in the scribbled grass, lies in the weak horizontal position, while the large vertical mother stands at the steps demanding that he come in from play. The art expresses the frustration of his diary entry, "My mom made me come in, so I couldn't play anymore."

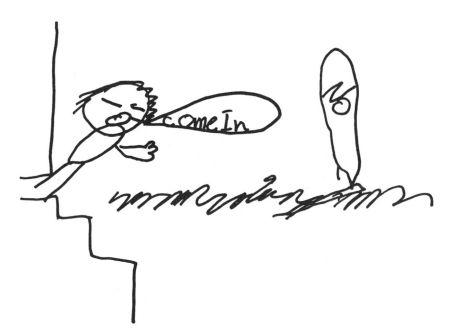

FIGURE 3. "My mom made me come in, so I couldn't play anymore."

A 10-year-old boy wrote about his eyeglasses as sources of stress for several days. Ironically, the subject of his eyeglasses did not appear in his parents' journals over the same time period. Repeated daily stressors included, "I lost my glasses. . . . I broke my glasses. . . . Today I fixed my own glasses. . . . I left my glasses at school. . . ." On the day of the drawing shown in Figure 4, highlighting the eyeglasses, his diary said, "Today I got new glasses. Now I have two pair." From the diary and drawing, we sense satisfaction, competence, control, and relief because he now has two pairs of eyeglasses.

Children's drawings, when compared with sibling and parental diaries, were especially helpful in understanding the family dynamics in a particular stressor situation. For example, a 9-year-old girl drew the picture in Figure 5. Her journal read, "I got kicked in the back at school. The best part of the day was that I got to ride in an ambulance. It was the first time I ever did." Her drawing is bright, with well-defined human figures and colorful detail. She has gold hair and is wearing a bright purple shirt, blue pants (both positive colors of health and spirit), and a well-labeled green oxygen mask. Her school and ambulance are also labeled, and the light on the ambulance shines with rays much like a happy sun. Three little blue flowers grace the door to the school. An arrow points to herself under the word "me," as if to say, "Look, this is me. I am having an adventure."

On the same day, shown in Figure 6, the drawing by her 11-year-old brother portrays quite a different image. Compare the figure of his sister with her own portrayal in Figure 5. In the brother's drawing, the figure of the girl is primitive, without color, detail, or expression, in a bleak, horizontal profile. Standing over her is another

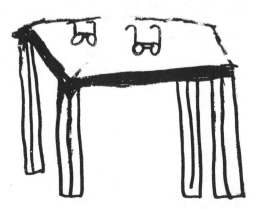

FIGURE 4. "Today I got new glasses. Now I have two pair."

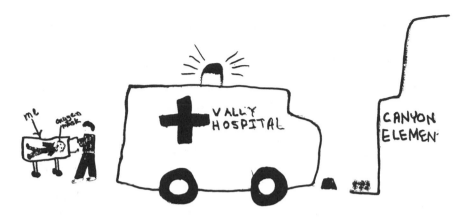

FIGURE 5. "I got kicked in the back at school. The best part of the day was that I got to ride in an ambulance. It was the first time I ever did."

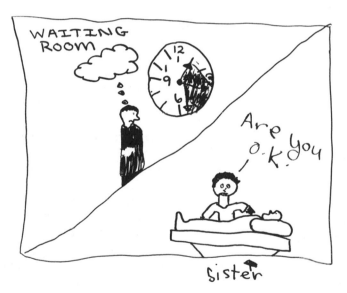

FIGURE 6. "My sister fell on a rock and hurt her back. She had to go to the hospital. I hope she will be O.K."

figure without color and with an expression of concern asking, "Are you O.K.?" A diagonal line separates the brother from his sister, as he waits in the marked waiting room with a distinct frown on his face and unexpressed images in his mind. To his side is a clock, larger than himself. Notice the difficulty with drawing the clock, marked by scribbled black lines. Combined with the label of the waiting room, this suggests a long wait and uncertainty about the condition of his sister and the time.

Further insights were found in the diaries of these two children and their mother over subsequent days. For the next 6 to 8 days, the emphasis in all three diaries was concern for the sister, even though she was released from the hospital without apparent serious injury. The sister showed evidence of enjoying the attention; she mentioned the ambulance experience, friends asking about her, and receiving presents. The mother noted the stressor of the event and how the sister was recovering, without mentioning the response of the brother. The brother expressed concern about his sister. From the drawings and the brother's diary, we learn that a significant invisible stress situation in the family during that time seemed to reside with the brother. It was he who apparently needed assurance and support, yet the focus of the entire family seemed to be upon the sister, who actually seemed to be adapting quite well.

The advantage of data collection over time is especially evident in Figures 7 and 8. Figure 7 is drawn by a 10-year-old boy on the day when he wrote, "No one would play with me. The best part of today was when I got to play flys [*sic*] up. They *let* me." Notice the dark, primitive nature of the human figures, which are all brown. The boy stands far in the upper left corner, at some distance from a mass of other figures apparently playing a game. The drawing is rather bleak, and elicits concern about the condition of the boy.

However, in Figure 8, we see another drawing on a different day by the same boy. On this day, a sun with rays appears in the center of the drawing. The figures are detailed and filled in with color, showing two boys playing football on green grass. The figure of the child's playmate is wearing a "healthy color" (Siegel, 1986, p. 160) blue shirt and brown pants, as he smiles and stretches his hands toward the ball and the boy. We see a figure of the child artist, the largest figure in the picture, in full uniform including helmet, with his name across his shirt, and red and blue stripes at the top of his socks. Verbal dialogue might have clarified why his own face is not drawn. Is there a problem, or does this just represent his portrayal of a complete uniform? His diary stated, "The best part of today was that I played football because I wanted to."

Notice the difference in perception of control. One day, "they *let* me play" and another day, "I played because I wanted to." This incident offers excellent evidence that the assessment of life stress in children (perhaps in adults too) must be made over time. If, for example, the

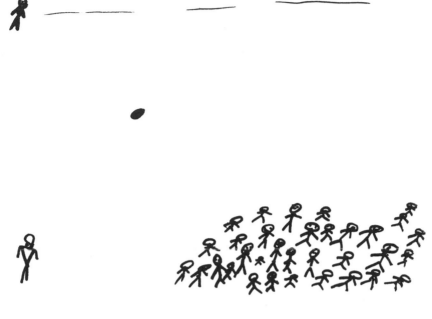

FIGURE 7. "No one would play with me. The best part of today was when I got to play flys [*sic*] up. They *let* me."

drawings of this boy were to be used in therapy or an assessment for litigation, one day's assessment would be quite different than the other, and could have critical implications. Indeed, when studying healthy people, changes over time may be more dynamic than in cases of pathology.

We are left to wonder about the motives and perceptions of the seven children in the study who did not offer a single drawing. We also have much to learn from the child who offered the happy drawing in Figure 9, who responded to the stressor of the first day of school, "I just went on with my life!" Flowers, green grass, raindrops, and rainbows, all typically positive images in the art of healthy children, were sprinkled throughout many of the diary entries in the study.

In this exploration, 49.8% of children's total diary entries were accompanied by a drawing. Boys produced 267 drawings, reflecting 50.0% of their total diary entries, and girls offered 349 pictures, representing 46.0% of their daily journal entries.

Table 9 shows the proportion of the children's drawing that obviously reflected and/or expanded corresponding written journal

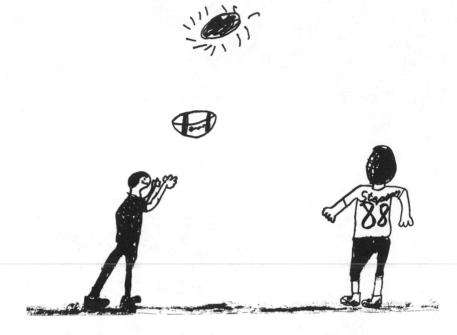

FIGURE 8. "The best part of today was that I played football because I wanted to."

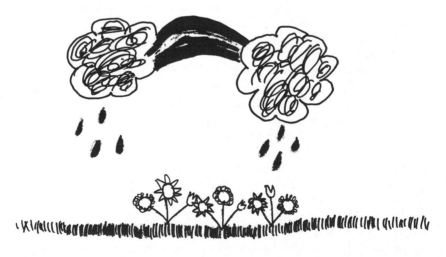

FIGURE 9. "I just went on with my life!"

TABLE 9. Proportion of Children's Art That Reflected Reported
Stress–Coping Experiences[a]

	Total (%)	Boys (%)	Girls (%)
Art portrayed reported stressor only	4.0	1.5	6.0
Art portrayed reported stressor and coping response	2.5	0.0	4.3
Art portrayed reported coping response only	1.9	4.1	0.0
Art portrayed reported uplifts/resources	20.4	19.5	21.2
Art did not seem directly related to reported stress-coping experience	71.2	74.9	68.5
TOTAL	100.0	100.0	100.0

[a]616 drawings; 267 from boys, 349 from girls.

entries for given days. The table indicates whether art work depicted
stressors, the entire stress–coping experience, coping responses, uplifts
or resources, or whether the drawings simply did not relate directly to
diary entries. Most drawings (71.2%) could not be associated with the
stated stress experiences without direct dialogue with the children.
However, art that related to expressed stress-coping perceptions was
particularly powerful in enriching the perspective.

As the table shows, when directly representing written entries,
children were most likely to draw uplift or resource experiences. It is
also interesting to note that girls seemed more likely to draw stressors,
whereas boys depicted coping situations.

Table 10 reflects children's use of color and written labels in the
art. The high proportion (40.8% total; boys, 50.9%; girls, 33.0%) of
the use of a single color may invalidate common assumptions that have
associated better emotional health with the more liberal use of color.

The liberal use of word labels, as children attempted to interpret
and explain their art, also testifies to children's ability and desire to
communicate their own world view.

TABLE 10. Use of Word Labels and Color in Children's Art

	Total (%)	Boys (%)	Girls (%)
Drawings in only one color	40.8	50.9	33.0
Multicolored drawings	59.3	49.1	67.1
TOTAL	100.1[a]	100	100.1
Used word labels to explain art	14.3	10.1	17.5

[a]Totals do not equal 100 due to rounding error.

Table 11 shows frequencies of children's art according to general content depicted. The area of human figures is broken down to show the frequencies of pictures in which children obviously depicted their own family members. Among the drawings of human figures, self representation was extremely common.

Symbols included single objects such as hearts, single objects, toys, and so forth. Abstractions often included colorful designs that did not seem to represent any objects in reality. Other topics are self-explanatory. Thought pictures included obvious deliberately imagined situations.

Girls most frequently drew human figures, whereas boys most often drew isolated symbols. Boys were more likely to draw outdoor play situations, indoor play, and vehicles (cars, trucks, tanks, etc.) than girls. Girls more frequently drew landscapes, flowers, and church or school situations.

Although less than one-third of the children's spontaneous art depicted the stress–coping experiences expressed in the diaries, the drawings were powerful in offering clarification and allowing the investigator into the child's world. Verbal dialogue with the children about their particular drawings might have further clarified the data.

The children's drawings in this study enriched the diary entries. They clarified written responses, and allowed a more complete picture of the child's reality. In some cases they gave powerful clues to

TABLE 11. Topics Depicted in Children's Art

	Total (%)	Boys (%)	Girls (%)
Human figures	23.6	15.4	29.8
(Total: family members or self)	(2.8)	(3.0)	(2.6)
Single symbols	19.0	25.5	14.0
Abstractions (designs)	11.9	10.9	12.6
Animals	8.6	9.0	8.3
Landscape without house	7.5	5.6	8.9
Scenes of outdoor play	7.0	9.7	4.9
Vehicles	4.4	7.9	1.7
Landscape with house	4.1	3.0	4.9
Flowers	3.3	2.3	4.0
Scenes of indoor play	3.1	4.5	2.0
Church/school activities	3.1	1.5	4.3
Fruits and vegetables	3.1	3.8	2.6
Thought pictures, dream-type images	1.6	1.1	2.0
TOTAL	100.3[a]	100.2	100.0

[a]Totals do not equal 100 due to rounding error.

meaning. In others the drawings contrasted with the written diary messages and a verbal exchange would have been helpful.

Future research would be enhanced by the use of both semistructured journals and drawings among all family members, including adults.

SUMMARY AND CONCLUSIONS

In considering the use of qualitative descriptive methods to reveal the world view of school-age children, original art must be recognized. Art has been called the language of children. The use of art in data collection, diagnosis, and therapy began with projective techniques from psychology. Subsequently, some psychometric instruments have been derived from objective criteria developed to evaluate particular drawing tasks. Recently, there has been more emphasis on the analysis of symbols in children's spontaneous drawings.

As scientific interest in children's art increases, ethical and validity concerns regarding intuitive interpretation arise. However, the significance of the meaning and enrichment offered by children's art seems to outweigh the weaknesses in objective measurement.

Art analysis and therapy have been used most with children who suffer trauma: terminal physical illness, mental illness, and abuse. Validation of symbolic meaning has mostly emerged from these populations. Validation among well children is meager.

This study offered the option of a daily drawing with colored markers. A few examples are described. Results showed that children's drawings can give helpful information regarding daily stress–coping phenomena, validated the importance of data collection over time, and reaffirmed the value of data from multiple family members. Drawings from these well children also validated some of the criteria for symbolic analysis previously applied to children in trauma. The use of art in this study demonstrated that children's art offers an effective and unobtrusive vehicle for obtaining meaningful descriptive qualitative data over time. The use of art as a means of data collection might effectively be expanded to include all family members.

Suggestions for Future Research and Clinical Practice

The study of stress–coping phenomena, particularly among children from within a family context, embraces multiple conceptual and empirical complexities. Such analysis implies the need for the identification and description of concepts and processes to derive valid theoretical foundations, and a naturalistic exploration of interrelated variables in order to accurately reflect empirical realities.

THEORETICAL PHILOSOPHY: INTEGRATION

The aim of this exploration was not to test or derive theory, but to empirically explore and describe concepts by which theory might be refined. Existing theory has contributed to conceptualization, approaches to data, and analysis, as well as to cognitive maps and perspectives for study. In Chapter 1, several possible perspectives for study of stress–coping phenomena were outlined. Subsequent chapters reviewed literature and reported research from several of those perspectives, including the individual perspective on individuals, which has been the traditional historical viewpoint for study; the family perspective on families, which represents a large body of family research, although unfortunately it has often omitted the subjective viewpoint of the child; and the child's and family's perspective on children. Whereas no single perspective is better or more comprehensive than another. It is a valuable exercise to recognize and acknowledge the perspective of study, so as not to make faulty assumptions about data sources and empirical applications, as sometimes happens.

Several theoretical viewpoints contributed to the exploration and conceptualization of study in this book. As discussed, these included symbolic interactionism, developmental theory, systems theory, and social exchange theory. In the study of stress and coping in children within the family setting, an integration of ABCX family stress theory and cognitive-phenomenological philosophy provided a particularly useful backdrop.

ABCX offers a model for viewing stress responses from a family perspective. However, it is enhanced by concepts from the cognitive-transactional viewpoint.

Children's daily stressors reported in this study might depict either the major stressor (A factor), pileups (aA factor, according to ABCX theory), or "hassles" (according to cognitive-transactional theory). Such conceptual distinctions still need to be clarified. Resources of uplifts found in this research probably represent more clearly the mediating variables described in cognitive-transactional theory than "bB factors" of family resources according to the ABCX model.

The cognitive-transactional concept of appraisal has emerged as essentially significant from child and parental viewpoints. Differences in perception within individuals over time and across different family members at the same time challenges some assumptions of ABCX theory about the "C factors" of family perception of particular stressor events.

The idea of cognitive adaptation (Taylor, 1983) was evident as children not only spontaneously reported intrapsychic stress-coping phenomena, but reported positive cognitive reframing in coping efforts. However, parental perception or synchrony with such processes in children was limited. The emerging resiliency model of family stress, adjustment, and adaptation (McCubbin & McCubbin, in press) may help to accommodate such issues from the perspective of the family.

Lazarus and Folkman (1984) cautioned against studying stressors and coping efforts without considering the interrelationships in the transaction between the individual and the environment, and asserted that coping strategies could not be accurately considered without viewing the entire process of related stressors, appraisal, and resources. Indeed, such processes must also be observed across individuals and family systems. Although the identification and classification of phenomena does contribute to knowledge, such reductionism can constitute an arbitrary assault on scientific integrity. Thus, categories must be assessed as they relate to each other and to the children and families.

Whereas this study attempted to explore the stress-coping process by examining both individual categories and relationships among those categories, further study is needed of such interrelationships. This research has shown the value of such exploration by observing subjects from their own individual perspective, in their natural setting over time, and in the context of the whole process rather than its fragmented parts. Observations were made on a daily basis of actual stressors and corresponding coping responses and resources, with parent–child comparisons within the family.

Methods

A major obstacle to discovering a child's perspective of reality was the achievement of a means of observation that was neither intrusive nor artificial. As noted, measures among children have traditionally been scaled-down revisions of adult instruments, or brief one-time interview encounters, which compromised the regard for the unique perspective of the child over time.

Coles (1990) noted in his own study of children:

> How does one learn from children. . . . I have no "survey research" to offer, nor am I interested in making generally psychological statements without reference to idiosyncrasies and exceptions. I do, though rely upon certain assumptions about children—that we as human beings possess awareness or consciousness, and that, through language, we try to understand the world around us and to convey what we have learned to other. . . . I stop well short of large-scale generalizations. (p. 22)

In selecting methods for this study, a major consideration was how to use a phenomenological, existential approach that would include all family members. Direct observation seemed to offer an incomplete behavioristic perspective, and interviewing seemed too artificial, unless sustained over many situations. The need was to somehow get inside the child's unique, private perspective. A daily, open-ended journal directed specifically toward pertinent variables seemed appropriate.

The use of diaries for data collection allowed for authentic, direct responses from the children over time. The semistructured, open-ended nature of the instruments allowed for directed observation of day-to-day phenomena from a child's perspective, without investigator intrusion. Diaries as a means of data collection also proved to be economical, in terms of time and resources, for retrieving broadly focused qualitative data. Diaries allowed the children to respond honestly without attempting to predict investigator expectations or relying on hypothetical situations, as might occur in isolated interview situations.

The children's drawings also enriched the survey of daily life and proved to be valuable in studying everyday life among well children. As noted, others cautioned that journal studies might produce a low rate of return and a high rate of attrition. However, in this study, even when children were told they need not make entries every day (in efforts to avoid the possibility of the research itself becoming the stressor), the children's responses exceeded the number of responses from the parents.

Although the semistructured journal proved to be effective in many ways, some significant limitations became evident. First, large volumes of qualitative data can challenge even the best systems for content analysis. For example, if only 30 subjects complete daily journals for a period of 6 weeks, responding to only five items (30 subjects, multiplied by 7 days, multiplied by 6 weeks, multiplied by five items), the total number of items requiring coding would be 6,300, each with contextual characteristics requiring investigator interpretation.

Another major limitation of the journals, as noted, was the inability to clarify or probe beyond the diary entries—as when, for example, I was unable to probe into the situation of the boy who wrote, "Everything went wrong today, so I kicked my sister." This problem reflects the potential strength of effective interviewing, although interview techniques as currently practiced may be inadequate for supporting critical articulation from a child, unless sustained, repeated over time, or achieved at the most timely moments of a child's daily life.

As an investigator, and fellow human being, I wondered about and longed to understand the meaning behind entries from the boy who wrote on several occasions, "No one will play with me . . . nothing was good, nothing was good." One day he reported the best part of the day to be, "Some boys *let* me play with them." Was he truly persecuted by his peers, and if so, why? or did he perceive himself as somehow unworthy to initiate peer relationships, and dependent upon friends' permission to relate? Impressions from daily art work seemed to shed light on some of these questions.

Did the rural boy who hid in a ditch, because he was afraid of some bulls, do so simply as a positive problem-solving response to a dangerous situation, or was he overtaken by personal fear and helplessness as he tried to avoid a constant, daily, misunderstood source of personal threat? Each of us as adults can remember an incident or a series of interactions that affected our self-esteem, instilled life-long fears, and influenced our behaviors, our perceptions of the world, indeed, our very sense of self. Yet such incidents may have been perceived as trivial by someone else. Indeed, many adults seek therapy to overcome the effects of such childhood transactions that become buried in life's clutter, yet continue to hurt.

To gain an understanding of such traumas, challenges, and human responses *as* they occur in childhood might open a door to sustained health through adulthood. Furthermore, we have much to learn from the joyful child who is able to appraise life's stressors as meaningful challenges, drawing health rather than pain from his or her existence, as, for instance, the child who reported on the first day of school, "Today was a super day!"

Methods must be refined and developed to reveal the meaning of a child's life experience from his or her own appraisal, with attention to individual differences. Such methods might include imagery, drawings, or games, but at the very least must include an investigator who is able to empathetically tune in to the child's perspective, spend the time needed to explore that perspective, and offer appropriate insight into its meaning. Perhaps therapy methods could be used for research and health education. There remains the fundamental challenge to develop methods for understanding cognitive–behavioral transactional processes in children.

There is also still much to be learned about the child's contribution to data obtained from families. When family coping and resources are studied, the child's view must be better integrated into the family equation. In this study, Knutson's comparison of parent–child data, which analyzed parental ability to perceive the concerns of the child, were a helpful contribution.

Data from children enhance the "family" perspective. For example, in this study, children reported many stressors reflecting disrupted family relationships, stressors induced by events related to family function or structure, or stressors otherwise related to family life. Furthermore, the family perspective was enriched by collecting data from several family members, with children's data as the primary focus.

It must be noted, even in this study that the problem of gaining data from all family members persists. Even when both parents were encouraged to submit written daily journals, the majority were offered by mothers, limiting the viewpoint.

MEANING OF THE DATA

The taxonomies derived from this study attempt to identify, organize, and refine the rich data on stress–coping phenomena obtained from children. A pervading theme in the children's diary responses was a realistic sense of their limited control over many daily life events. It is significant that the most common coping response to actual daily stressors was submission or endurance.

Among the interpersonal responses, the children's mothers were reported as the most common source of social support. This validated a common finding in various areas of family study (Ferree, 1990; Fowlkes, 1980). The relative absence of the father as a perceived source of support is an issue meriting further study.

The differences between parent and child perceptions provide clues about the realities of family communication. Parents perceived themselves as the source of the children's stress more than the children indicated. Parents showed little awareness of children's concerns regarding family members and issues. Parents also seemed to misread the stressors of extracurricular activities and some intrapsychic sources of stress. Generally, parents noticed the behavioral manifestations of children's stress–coping processes, but seemed relatively unaware of cognitive and emotional coping responses. Perhaps this is because behavioral responses are more visible. It seems that parenting education, which has traditionally been focused on behavior, ought also to help parents be aware of children's cognitive/emotional experiences.

Gender differences are apparent in reports of stress–coping experiences, as evidenced by the frequencies among categories of the taxonomies. Girls were more likely to identify emotional-sensory and emotional-expression coping responses than boys. Boys were more likely to use physical aggression in coping. As coping resources, girls reported more social support and intrapsychic comfort, whereas boys led in physical–social activities and physical comfort. These findings are consistent with other research, including the inductive studies of Walker (1988) and Ryan (1989).

Analysis

Coles (1990) warned of the need for restraint in the scientific drive to order and graphically model phenomena about children. Our propensity is to "grab for conclusions and interpretations, to rush to classify." Coles continued that:

> "Data" are too often offered to us with no warnings about the limits of their usefulness . . . with no context given for what is being handed down as truth. (p. 22)

By its very nature, the inductive approach of content analysis addresses categories, or fragments, of processes, in order to explore and theorize regarding the larger process perspective. Methods of analysis in this research attempted to decrease the fragmented reductionism of categories.

Although there are some computer programs for qualitative data management (Fielding & Lee, 1991; Tesch, 1987), most of these are based on *word* rather than *context* reductions. Because such programs manage, rather than analyze, data, investigator sensitivity to the meaning of data is critical.

In transactional processes, there is a risk of losing the nuances of meaning in situation-or process-dependent responses. For example, one child in this study listed homework as a stressor. Depending on other contextual information, this could have been appraised as distaste for the chore itself, an allusion to a sense of personal responsibility over not getting the work done or forgetting the assignment, a sense of internal discomfort about not understanding the teacher expectations, or annoyance at the generally confining atmosphere of school.

Another example is the coping response of "playing with friends," which could relate to an attempt at distraction, or to the interpersonal focus of a particular relationship. When subjects listed "trying to make friends" as a coping response, it may have reflected an active problem-solving approach to the challenge of the first day of school, or it may have been behavioral reframing in response to the stress of "a friend is not nice to me." Such nuances, strongly related to context and individual appraisal, had to be determined from the complete background of daily diary entries. Thus, although coding and analysis showed a high degree of reliability, the validity of taxonomies is still in question. Now that several similar inductive taxonomies of children's stressors and coping are emerging in the literature, it would be helpful to perform a meta-analysis on all taxonomies developed to date.

Even when considering personal context, one must assess whether content analysis is the only appropriate means for qualitative analysis. Taxonomy construction is recognized as an effective and broadly accepted method for managing volumes of qualitative data from a grounded theory approach. The themes and categories emerging from this particular investigation offer a new knowledge base, as well as a unique quantitative perspective based on the frequencies and other descriptive presentations. However, in such quantitative reduction, there is a risk that qualitative data may appear poorly assimilated or contrived, without portraying the richness and nuance of individual observations. Perhaps a purely phenomenological narrative offering of vignettes from the children, or case study reports would have been as effective.

Development of Taxonomies

Several authors (Folger et al., 1984; Garvin et al., 1987) have advocated the development of taxonomies with small, concrete, exhaustive categories in order to ensure validity, reliability, and a secure foundation upon which to build further study.

The development in this study of a few conceptual themes among stressors, coping responses, and coping resources provided a general perspective and allowed for the manageability of multiple data for discussion. However, the numerous categories were not reduced further than presented because of their value for current and future research, which may identify similarities and patterns for reduction. A variety of categories further provides an exhaustive foundation for the identification of variables when developing instruments to measure stress appraisal or coping styles. Instruments which are based on actual subject perception have not yet been developed. The few broad themes of this study can be scrutinized and tested, and may make a contribution to theory. The unwieldiness of the many categories that emerged here may be tolerated as a first step along the path of theory refinement and measurement development.

This exploration offered information beyond the simple narrative description and categorization provided by previous qualitative studies. The frequency tables provided the proportions of responses in various categories and the numerical relationships among variables. This kind of data presentation and interpretation provides a foundation for constructing and testing hypotheses, and could be used for the development of profile descriptions in instrument development and standardization.

QUALITATIVE RESEARCH WITH CHILDREN

The assumptions listed in Chapter 4 were validated by observing children in the family setting. Although pilot study participants and clinicians, and others warned of children's limited linguistic articulation or willingness to comply in a longitudinal diary study, the children overwhelmingly performed beyond expectations.

Parents of this study had relatively high level of education, and Steeves and Bostian (1982) observed diary compliance to be positively related to level of education. Concerns regarding diary compliance over time (Steeves & Bostian, 1982) among children were invalidated. Indeed, diary compliance among the children was 9% higher than among parents.

The children showed a remarkable intuitive sense of abandon and a willingness to share themselves in both the written responses and the art. They needed little instruction and asked few questions, yet provided appropriate, rich data.

Individual appraisal was a key factor that significantly influenced the analysis of the transactions. The types of stressor appraisals listed by Folkman and Lazarus (1984) of harm–loss, threat, challenge, and simple annoyance were evident across all categories. Indeed, as proposed by Lazarus (1981), appraisal seemed to be the chief determining variable in coping responses to a given stressor.

Unfortunately, no effort was made to address appraisal from a perspective of time, for example, in short- versus long-term transactions. For example, some children responded to the perceived stressors of the immediate situation, such as forgetting homework, whereas others mentioned long-term concerns, such as worries about family finances. The consistency of particular stressors over time versus episodic stressors was not explored. Such information is critical in evaluating and intervening in specific individual and family situations. The factor of individual appraisal needs to be understood in order to be able to identify effective responses to particular stressors or to particular patterns of coping responses.

CONCLUSIONS AND RECOMMENDATIONS

The need for further study has already been pointed out in several areas. My hope is that results of this research will contribute to (1) further descriptive exploration, (2) hypothesis generation and testing, and (3) education, guidance, and therapy grounded in data from children and families.

Future Exploration

This study, which employed a fairly uncommon method for data collection, broadened the field of possible means of observing children from their own perspective. Effective replication of results might be achieved by diaries and other modified creative approaches to data collection and analysis. Further longitudinal study might employ diaries, ethnographic interviews, imagery, or various means of artistic expression as techniques of data collection. Data could be presented by categorization, comparative analysis, quantification, or case study methods. There is ultimately a need to develop and test instruments sensitive to children's perceptions and realities, and theory related to stress appraisal and coping styles, with the subsequent identification and prediction of stress–coping profiles among children.

It is important to include data from all family members, and to integrate the type of information obtained in this study into the entire family equation. More data are needed regarding the typical living situations of children and families. As the science develops interventions, the evaluation of those interventions is heavily dependent upon baseline data regarding subjective perceptions and individual differences.

Robins (1983) noted that "single dramatic life events are, by definition, time-limited and differ from one's typical living situation" (p. 336). Although much of our research and clinical practice must be directed at helping people survive major trauma—such as illness, death, divorce—more information is needed about the maintenance and promotion of health, and daily life adaptation. In children and families who live with chronic adversity (such as poverty, chronic illness, or dysfunctional social relationships), there is a need to study the possible potentiating effects of superimposed daily hassles and associated coping efforts.

Such study also needs to be replicated for and expanded into populations of differing cultural background, race, socioeconomic status, age, and condition of life, such as among ill people or people undergoing particular life trauma. Before valid instrument or therapy development can be achieved, the refinement and validation of naturalistic studies such as these must be accomplished.

There is a need to expand our models to include a comprehensive list of significant variables in the stress–coping transaction. Social scientists tend to exclude physiological factors. For example, in development of the Feel Bad Scale, Lewis and associates (1984) excluded children's reports of stressors that produced physical discomfort, such as feeling sick. Physiological variables must be included for a holistic approach. Research must move beyond the traditional correlation studies, described in Chapter 1 and Chapter 3, that associate major life events with physical symptoms. Effects of daily life stress and of chronic stressors overtime on physiological processes, such as endocrine responses, also need to be examined. For example, Hanson and Pichert (1986) observed that everyday stress in diabetic children was directly related to the control of blood sugar levels.

Model expansion must come from multidisciplinary research efforts. Adams (1988) noted the general movement in family research to be "cross-disciplinary, cross-institutional, and cross-cultural," in order to "take the old conceptual frameworks forward to new insights" (p. 17).

Generating Research Questions

Since the purpose of this study was exploration, the questions generated, even from these data, were not tested. Research questions meriting further study include the following: (1) Are stress and coping phenomena consistent among families? (2) Are stress and coping phenomena consistent within individual subjects? (3) Are there differences in stress–coping patterns among children of various cultural backgrounds, including ethnic, rural, suburban? (4) What is the meaning of the differences between parents and children in reports of stress–coping patterns? (5) What are the relationships among the content of drawings and stress–coping patterns? (6) What are the relationships between stressor categories and coping categories?

Other research questions generated include the following: (1) What are the daily stress–coping phenomena among children undergoing particular (acute and/or chronic) stressful situations? (2) Which coping responses are most effective? (3) What are the differences between children who employ consistency in coping responses and those who employ a large repertoire of coping strategies? (4) How do gender or developmental status affect stress–coping phenomena? (5) Can effective coping responses be learned? (6) Do individual appraisal and/or coping patterns change as life situations change? (7) How do daily stress–coping phenomena differ between well children and ill children?

As these and other questions are answered, subsequent research questions might include: (1) What are the most effective methods to teach children effective appraisal and coping? (2) How can the quality and duration of life and health be enhanced by guidance in effective appraisal and coping? Rutter (1983) noted:

> Not only do we have to ask whether the processes involved in stress and coping differ according to the child's stage of development, but more particularly we need to determine whether adverse experiences or hap-

penings [as well as coping responses] alter the course of subsequent development or influence the ways in which an individual responds to much later stress events." (p. 2)

Family Education, Guidance, and Therapy

Although the results of this investigation generated more questions than answers, some light was shed on how to intervene with families. The critical need for an empathetic approach to the child, in order to obtain valid data for research or therapy, was underscored. Means to reach children unobtrusively were demonstrated; diaries could be employed in family education and therapy. The research validated that children are capable of self-expression, and willing and eager for self-discovery, and that data may be drawn from both children and parents.

The various categories of stressors and coping responses may be observed and validated among children in education, guidance, and care. A knowledge of the categories and themes help those who teach or guide children to understand stressors and promote coping repertoires. Educators and clinicians may now have a clearer picture of the nature of stressors and responses, and the differences in parent and child appraisal. Presumably, such knowledge will contribute to a more empathetic understanding of families.

As Wright and Leahey (1987) noted, interactions in families must be observed over time. The variable of the passage of time in everyday life is crucial to revealing meaning in the links and patterns of family life. When clinically intervening with families, it is also important to know when it is best to direct treatment toward changing the stressor, helping to alter appraisal or perceptions, or helping to enhance and evaluate coping efforts.

This research validated the findings (Band & Weisz, 1988) that reports of coping behavior are not confined to children facing extraordinary kinds of stress, and that children as young as 6 or 7 years are

> sufficiently aware of stress and coping in their own lives to report conditions and events that they find stressful, describe their own efforts to coping, and evaluate the efficacy of those efforts. (p. 253)

Given an effective vehicle, it is evident from this exploration that children can articulate private perceptions, that data can be drawn from more than one family member, and that subjective reports from well people can offer valuable information.

R E F E R E N C E S

Achenbach, T. M., & Edelbrock, C. (1981). *Child behavior checklist for ages 4–16.* Burlington, VT: University of Vermont.

Adams, B. N. (1986). *The family: A sociological interpretation* (4th ed.). San Diego: Harcourt Brace Jovanovich.

Adams, B. N. (1988). Fifty years of family research: What does it mean? *Journal of Marriage and the Family, 50,* 5–17.

Aiken, S. (1982). Family structure and utilization of cancer support groups. *Oncology Nursing Forum, 9,* 22–26.

Aldous, J. (1990). Family development and the life course: Two perspectives on family change. *Journal of Marriage and the Family, 52,* 571–583.

Altshuler, J. L., & Ruble, D. N. (1989). Developmental changes in children's awareness of strategies for coping with uncontrollable stress. *Child Development, 60,* 1337–1349.

Amato, P. R., & Ochiltree, G. (1987). Interviewing children about their families: A note on data quality. *Journal of Marriage and the Family, 49,* 669–675.

Angell, R. O. (1936). *The family encounters the Depression.* New York: Scribner.

Anthony, E. J. (1991). The response to overwhelming stress in children: Some introductory comments. In A. Monat & R. S. Lazarus (Eds.), *Stress and coping: An anthology* (3rd ed., pp. 307–318). New York: Columbia University Press.

Anthony, E. J., & Cohler, B. J. (Eds.). (1987). *The invulnerable child.* New York: Guilford Press.

Antonovsky, A. (1979). *Health, stress, and coping.* San Francisco: Jossey-Bass.

Appley, M. H., & Trumbull, R. (Eds). (1986). *Dynamics of stress: Physiological, Psychological, and Social Perspectives.* New York: Plenum Press.

Atkins, F. D. (1991). Children's perspective of stress and coping: An integrative review. *Issues in Mental Health Nursing, 12,* 171–178.

Auerbach, S. M., Martelli, M. F., & Mercuri, L. G. (1983). Anxiety, information, interpersonal impacts, and adjustment to a stressful health care situation. *Journal of Personality and Social Psychology, 44,* 1284–1296.

Austin, J. K., Patterson, J. M., & Huberty, T. J. (1991). Development of the

Coping Health Inventory for Children. *Journal of Pediatric Nursing, 6,* 166–174.

Bach, S. (1966). Spontaneous paintings of severely ill patients. *Acta Psychosomatica, 8,* 1–66.

Bach, S. (1975). Spontaneous drawings of leukemic children as an expression of the total personality, mind and body. *Acta Paedopsychiatrica, 41,* 86–104.

Baker, S. R. (1991). Utilizing art and imagery in death and dying counseling. In D. Papadotou & C. Papadatos (Eds.), *Children and death* (pp. 161–175). New York: Hemisphere.

Baldwin, C. (1977). *One to one: Self understanding through journal writing.* New York: M. Evans.

Ball, D., McKenry, P. C., & Price-Bonham, S. (1983). Use of repeated-measures designs in family research. *Journal of Marriage and the Family, 43,* 885–896.

Band, E. B., & Weisz, J. R. (1988). How to feel better when it feels bad: Children's perspectives on coping with everyday stress. *Developmental Psychology, 24,* 247–253.

Bargagliotti, L. A., & Trygstad, L. N. (1987). Differences in stress and coping findings: A reflection of social realities or methodologies? *Nursing Research, 36,* 170–173.

Barnes, L. B. (1988). Depressed and nondepressed children under stress: Their cognitive appraisals and coping responses. *Dissertation Abstracts International, 50,* 339-B (Order No. DA8901272).

Bedell, J. R., Giordani, B., Armour, J. L., Tavormina, J., & Boll, T. (1977). Life stress and the psychological and medical adjustment of chronically ill children. *Journal of Psychosomatic Research, 21,* 237–242.

Behr, S. K., Murphy, D. L., & Summers, J. A. (1992). *Kansas inventory of parental perceptions.* Wichita: University of Kansas.

Belenky, M. F., Clinchy, B. M., Goldberger, N. R., & Tarule, J. M. (1986). *Women's ways of knowing.* New York: Basic.

Belle, D. (1987). Gender differences in the social moderators of stress. In R. C. Barnett, L. Biener, & G. K. Baruch (Eds.), *Gender and stress* (pp. 257–277). New York: Free Press.

Belle, D. (1991). Gender differences in the social moderators of stress. In A. Monat & R. S. Lazarus (Eds.), *Stress and coping: An anthology* (3rd ed., pp. 258–274). New York: Columbia University Press.

Bem, S. (1983). Gender-schema theory and its implications for child development. *Signs, 8,* 598–616.

Bertalanffy, R. H. (1950). The theory of open systems in physics and biology. *Science, 111,* 23–29.

Bertalanffy, R. H. (1968). *General systems theory.* New York: George Braziller.

Bertaux, D. (1981). *Biography and society.* Beverly Hills, CA: Sage.

Beutler, I. F., Burr, W. R., Bahr, K. S., & Herrin, D. A. (1989). The family realm: Theoretical contributions for understanding its uniqueness. *Journal of Marriage and the Family, 51,* 805–816.

Bieliauskas, L. A. (1982). *Stress and its relationship to health and illness.* Boulder, CO: Westview Press.

Bishop, E. G., Hailey, B. J., & Anderson, H. N. (1987). Assessment of Type A behavior in children: A comparison of two instruments. *Journal of Human Stress, 13,* 121–127.

Blomeyer, R. (1978). Drawings of children during initial interviews as unconsciously determined by the interviewers. *Analytische Psychologie, 9,* 213–232.

Bluestein, V. (1978). Loss of loved ones and the drawing of dead or broken branches on the HTP. *Psychology in the Schools, 15,* 364–366.

Bobo, J. K., Gilchrist, L. D., Elmer, J. F., Snow, W. H., & Schinke, S. P. (1986). Hassles, role strain, and peer relations in young adolescents. *Journal of Early Adolescence, 6,* 339–352.

Bolger, N., DeLongis, A., Kessler, R. C., & Wethington, E. (1989). The contagion of stress across multiple roles. *Journal of Marriage and the Family, 51,* 175–183.

Boss, P. G. (1980a). The relationship of psychological father presence, wife's personal qualities, and wife/family dysfunction in families of missing fathers. *Journal of Marriage and the Family, 42,* 541–549.

Boss, P. G. (1980b). Normative family stress: Family boundary changes across the life-span. *Family Relations, 29,* 445–450.

Boss, P. G. (1983). The marital relationship: Boundaries and ambiguities. In C. Figley & H. I. McCubbin (Eds.), *Stress and the family* (Vol. 2). New York: Brunner/Mazel.

Boss, P. G. (1987). Family stress. In S. Sussman & S. Steinmetz (Eds.), *Handbook on marriage and the family* (pp. 695–723). New York: Plenum Press.

Boss, P. G. (1988). *Family stress management.* Beverly Hills, CA: Sage.

Bossert, E. A. (1990). The influence of health status, gender, and anxiety on the stress and coping processes of hospitalized school-age children. *Dissertation Abstracts International, 52,* 746-B (Order No. DA9119593).

Boyce, T. W., Jensen, E. W., Cassell, J. C., Collier, A. M., Smith, A. H., & Ramey, C. T. (1977). Influence of life events and family routines on childhood respiratory tract illness. *Pediatrics, 60,* 609–615.

Boyd, H. F., & Johnson, G. O. (1981). *Analysis of coping style.* Columbus, OH: Charles Merrill.

Brandell, J. R. (1986). Autogenic stories and projective drawings: Tools for the clinical assessment and treatment of severely disturbed and at-risk children. *Journal of Independent Social Work, 1,* 19–32.

Briggs, F., & Lehmann, K. (1989). Significance of children's drawings in cases of sexual abuse. *Early Child Development and Care, 47,* 131–147.

Brink, P. (1987). On reliability and validity in qualitative research. *Western Journal of Nursing Research, 9,* 157–159.

Brod, J. (1982). Introduction. In J. Bahlmann & H. Liebau (Eds.), *Stress and hypertension* (pp. 1–6). New York: Karger.

Broderick, C. B. (Ed.). (1971). *A decade of family research and action, 1960–1970.* Minneapolis: National Council on Family Relations.

Brown, J. M., O'Keeffe, J., Sanders, S. H., & Baker, B. (1986). Developmental changes in children's cognition to stressful and painful situations. *Journal of Pediatric Psychology, 11,* 343–345.

Brown, L. P., & Cowen, E. L. (1988). Children's judgments of event upsettingness and personal experiencing of stressful events. *American Journal of Community Psychology, 16,* 123–135.

Brumback, R. A. (1977). Characteristics of the Inside-of-the-Body test drawings performed by normal school children. *Perceptual Motor Skills, 44,* 703–708.

Bryant, B. K. (1985). The neighborhood walk, sources of support in middle childhood. *Monographs of the Society for Research on Child Development, 50,* 1–12.

Burgess, E. W. (1926). The family as a unity of interacting personalities. *The Family, 7,* 3–9.

Burr, R. G., Burr, W. R., & Holman, T. B. (in press). A systems model of family stress. In W. R. Burr & S. Klein (Eds.), *Managing family stress.* Newbury Park, CA: Sage.

Burr, W. R. (1973). *Theory construction and the sociology of the family.* New York: Wiley.

Burr, W. R., Herrin, D. A., Day, R. D., Beutler, I. F., & Leigh, G. K. (1988). Epistemologies that lead to primary explanations in family science. *Family Science Review, 1,* 185–210.

Burr, W. R., Hill, R., Nye, F. I., & Reiss, J. L. (Eds.). (1979). *Contemporary theories about the family: Vol. 1. Research based theories.* New York: Free Press.

Burr, W. R., Leigh, G. K., Day, R. D., & Constantine, J. (1979). Symbolic interaction and the family. In W. R. Burr, R. Hill, F. I. Nye., & I. L. Reiss (Eds.), *Contemporary theories about the family.* (Vol. 2). New York: Free Press.

Butz, A. M., & Alexander, C. (1991). Use of health diaries with children. *Nursing Research, 40,* 59–61.

Buxton, A. (1982, September). *Children's journals: Further dimensions of assessing language development.* Paper presented to North Dakota Study Group on Evaluation, Grand Forks, ND.

Call, E. T. (1983). The relationship between the perception of stress associated with life change, perception of autonomic response, and physical symptoms in children. *Dissertation Abstracts International, 45,* 343B. (University Microfilms No. DA840928)

Cannon, W. B. (1932). *The wisdom of the body.* New York: Norton.

Caplan, G. (1976). Mastery of stress: Psychosocial aspects. *American Journal of Psychiatry, 138,* 413–420.

Caplan, R. D., Naidu, R. K., & Tripathi, R. C. (1984). Coping and defense: Constellations versus components. *Journal of Health and Social Behavior, 25,* 303–320.

Case, C., & Dalley, T. (Eds.). (1990). *Working with children in art therapy.* London: Tavistock/Routledge.

Cassel, J. (1976). The contribution of the social environment to host resistance. *American Journal of Epidemiology, 104,* 107–123.

Caty, S., Ellerton, M. L., & Ritchie, J. A. (1984). Coping in hospitalized children: An analysis of published case studies. *Nursing Research, 33,* 277–282.

Chandler, L. A. (1981). The source of stress inventory. *Psychology in the Schools, 18,* 164–168.

Chandler, L. A. (1985). *Children under stress* (2nd ed.). Springfield, IL: Charles C. Thomas.

Chandler, L. A., & Johnson, V. J. (1991). *Using projective techniques with children: A guide to clinical assessment.* Springfield, IL: Charles C. Thomas.

Clements, I. W., & Roberts, F. B. (1983). *Family health: A theoretical approach to nursing care.* New York: Wiley.

Cobb, S. (1976). Social support as a moderator of life stress. *Psychosomatic Medicine, 38,* 300–314.

Coddington, R. D. (1972). The significance of life events as etiologic factors in disease of children. *Journal of Psychosomatic Research, 16,* 7–18.

Coelho, G. V., Hamberg, D. A., & Adams, J. E. (Eds.). (1974). *Coping and adaptation.* New York: Basic.

Cohen, D. S. (1985). Pediatric cancer: Predicting sibling adjustment. *Dissertation Abstracts International, 46,* 637. (University Microfilms No. ADG85-08044, 8508)

Cohen, F. (1982). Personality, stress, and the development of physical illness. In G. C. Stone, F. Cohen, & N. E. Adler (Eds.), *Health psychology: A handbook* (pp. 77–113). San Francisco: Jossey-Bass.

Cohen, F. W., & Phelps, R. E. (1985). Incest markers in children's artwork. *Arts in Psychotherapy, 12,* 165–283.

Cohen, M. Z. (1987). A historical overview of the phenomenologic movement. *Image: Journal of Nursing Scholarship, 19,* 31–34.

Cohen, S., & Wills, T. (1985). Stress, social support, and the buffering hypothesis. *Psychology Bulletin, 98,* 310–357.

Colaizzi, P. (1978). Psychological research as the phenomenologist views it. In R. Valle & M. King (Eds.), *Existential–phenomenological alternatives for psychology.* New York: Oxford University Press.

Coles, R. (1990). *The spiritual life of children.* Boston: Houghton Mifflin.

Colton, J. A. (1985). Childhood stress: Perceptions of children and professionals. *Journal of Psychopathology and Behavioral Assessment, 7,* 155–173.

Combrinck-Graham, L. (Ed.). (1988). *Children in family contexts: Perspectives on treatment.* New York: Guilford Press.

Compas, B. E., Davis, G. E., Forsythe, C. J., & Wagner, B. M. (1987). Assessment of major and daily stressful events during adolescence: The Adolescent Perceived Events Scale. *Journal of Consulting and Clinical Psychology, 55,* 534–541.

Compas, B. E., Malcarne, V. L., & Fondacaro, K. M. (1988). Coping with stressful events in older children and young adolescents. *Journal of Consulting and Clinical Psychology, 56,* 405–411.

Cooper, C. L. (Ed.). (1983). *Stress research: Issues for the eighties*. New York: Wiley.

Cooper, P. J., Bawden, H. N., Camfield, P. R., & Camfield, C. S. (1987). Anxiety and life events in childhood migraine. *Pediatrics, 79,* 999–1004.

Coopersmith, S., Sakai, D., Beardslee, B., & Coopersmith, A. (1976). Figure drawing as an expression of self-esteem. *Journal of Personality Assessment, 40,* 370–375.

Corbin, J. M., & Strauss, A. L. (1984). Collaboration: Couples working together to manage chronic illness. *Image: Journal of Nursing Scholarship, 14,* 109–115.

Cousins, N. (1976). Anatomy of an illness (as perceived by the patient). *New England Journal of Medicine, 295,* 1458–1463.

Cox, M. (1991). *The child's point of view* (2nd ed.). New York: Guilford Press.

Crnic, K. A., & Booth, C. L. (1991). Mothers' and fathers' perceptions of daily hassles of parenting across early childhood. *Journal of Marriage and the Family, 53,* 1042–1050.

Crnic, K. A., & Greenberg, M. T. (1990). Minor parenting stresses with young children. *Child Development, 61,* 1628–1637.

Curran, D. (1983). *Traits of a healthy family.* New York: Ballantine.

Curran, D. (1985). *Stress and the healthy family.* Minneapolis: Winston Press.

Curtis, J. D., & Detert, R. A. (1981). *How to relax: A holistic approach to stress management.* Palo Alto, CA: Mayfield.

Dalley, T., Case, C., Schaverien, J., Weir, F., Halliday, D., Halla, P. N., & Waller, D. (1987). *Images of art therapy: New developments in theory and practice.* London: Tavistock/Routledge.

Davison, G. C., & Neal, J. M. (1990). *Abnormal psychology* (5th ed.). New York: Wiley.

Deatrick, J. A., & Faux, S. A. (1991). Conducting qualitative studies with children and adolescents. In J. M. Morse (Ed.), *Qualitative nursing research: A contemporary dialogue* (pp. 203–223). Newbury Park, CA: Sage.

Delgorgue, M., & Engelhart, D. (1984). Style graphique chez l'enfant: Deux recherches sur la discrimination entre dessin d'enfant "normal" et dessin d'enfant "pathologique" [Graphic style among children: Two studies of differences between the drawings of "normal" and "pathological" children]. *Bulletin de Psychologie, 38,* 303–321.

DeLongis, A., Coyne, J. C., Dakof, G., Folkman, S., & Lazarus, R. S. (1982). Relationship of daily hassles, uplifts, and major life events to health status. *Health Psychology, 1,* 119–136.

DeMaio-Esteves, M. (1990). Mediators of daily stress and perceived health status in adolescent girls. *Nursing Research, 39,* 360–364.

Dennis, K. E. (1986). Q methodology: Relevance and application to nursing research. *Advances in Nursing Science, 8,* 6–17.

Denzin, N. K. (1973). *The research act: A theoretical introduction to sociological methods.* Chicago: Aldine.

Denzin, N. K. (1983). Interpretive interactionism. In G. Morgan (Ed.), *Beyond method: Strategies for social research* (pp. 129–146). Beverly Hills, CA: Sage.

DeWine, S. (1977, December). *Student journals in the communication classroom: A content analysis.* Paper presented at the Annual Meeting of the Speech Communication Association, Washington, DC.

Dibrell, L. L., & Yamamoto, K. (1988). In their own words: Concerns of young children. *Child Psychiatry and Human Development, 19,* 14–25.

Dickey, J. P., & Henderson, P. (1989). What young children say about stress and coping in school. *Health Education, February/March,* 14–17.

DiLeo, J. (1970). *Young children and their drawings.* New York: Brunner/Mazel.

DiLeo, J. (1983). *Interpreting children's drawings.* Brunner/Mazel.

Dise-Lewis, J. E. (1984). The assessment of stress in children: Development of the life events and coping inventory. *Dissertation Abstracts International, 45,* 667B. (University Microfilms No. DA8411928)

Dise-Lewis, J. E. (1988). The life events and coping inventory: An assessment of stress in children. *Psychosomatic Medicine, 50,* 484–499.

Dollahite, D. C. (1991). Family resource management and family stress theories: Toward a conceptual integration. *Lifestyles: Family and economic issues, 12,* 361–377.

Dollahite, D. C., & Winterhoff, P. A. (1992, November). *Individual and family temperament as mediators of adaptive behavior in a model of crisis/stress management.* Paper presented at National Council of Family Relations Theory Construction and Research Methodology Preconference Workshop, Orlando, FL.

Draper, T. W., & Marcos, A. C. (Eds.). (1990). *Family variables.* Newbury Park, CA: Sage.

Drew, N. (1986). Exclusion and confirmation: A phenomenology of patients' experiences with caregivers. *Image: Journal of Nursing Scholarship, 18,* 39–43.

Drotar, D., & Crawford, P. (1985). Psychological adaptation of siblings of chronically ill children: Research and practice implications. *Journal of Developmental Behavioral Pediatrics, 6,* 355–356.

Dubow, E. F., & Tisak, J. (1989). The relation between stressful life events and adjustment in elementary school children: The role of social support and social problem-solving skills. *Child Development, 60,* 1412–1423.

Dubow, E. F., Tisak, J., Causey, D., Hryshko, A., & Reid, G. (1991). A two-year longitudinal study of stressful life events, social support, and social problem-solving skills: Contributions to children's behavioral and academic adjustment. *Child Development, 62,* 583–599.

Dunn, J. (1985). *Sisters and brothers: The developing child.* Cambridge, MA: Harvard University Press.

Dunn, J., & Kendrick, C. (1982). Temperamental differences, family relationships, and young children's response to change within the family. *Ciba Foundation Symposium, 89,* 87–105.

Dunn, J., Kendrick, C., & MacNamee, R. (1981). The reaction of first-born children to the birth of a sibling: Mothers' reports. *Journal of Child Psychology and Psychiatry, 22,* 1–18.

Duvall, E. M. (1957). *Family development.* Philadelphia: Lippincott.

Eagleston, J. R., Kirmil-Gray, K., Thoresen, C. E., Widenfield, S. A., Bracke, P., Heft, L., & Arnow, B. (1986). Physical health correlates of Type A behavior in children and adolescents. *Journal of Behavioral Medicine, 9,* 341–362.

Elias, J. J., Gara, M., Ubriaco, M., Rothbaum, P. A., Clabby, J. F., & Schuyler, T. (1986). Impact of a preventive social problem-solving intervention on children's coping with middle-school stressors. *American Journal of Community Psychology, 14,* 259–275.

Elkind, D. (1981). *The hurried child.* Reading, MA: Addison-Wesley.

Elwood, S. W. (1987). Stressor and coping response inventories for children. *Psychological Reports, 60,* 931–947.

Englehardt, L. (1986, March). *Educational applications of biofeedback.* Paper presented at the 17th Annual Meeting of the Biofeedback Society of America, San Francisco, CA.

Epstein, N. B., Baldwin, L. M., & Bishop, D. S. (1983). The McMaster family assessment device. *Journal of Marital and Family Therapy, 9,* 171–180.

Erickson, E. H. (1963). *Childhood and society* (2nd ed.). New York: Norton.

Failla, S., & Jones, L. C. (1991). Families of children with developmental disabilities: An examination of family hardiness. *Research in Nursing and Health, 14,* 41–50.

Falk, J. D. (1981). Understanding children's art: An analysis of the literature. *Journal of Personality Assessment, 45,* 465–472.

Fawcett, J. (1975). The family as a living open system: An emerging conceptual framework for nursing. *International Nursing Review, 22,* 113–116.

Feetham, S. L. (1984). Family research: Issues and directions for nursing. In H. Werley & J. J. Fitzpatrick (Eds.), *Annual review of nursing research* (pp. 3–25). New York: Springer.

Felner, R. D. (1984). Vulnerability in childhood. In M. C. Roberts & L. Peterson (Eds.), *Prevention of problems in childhood* (pp. 133–169). New York: Wiley.

Ferree, M. M. (1990). Beyond separate spheres: Feminism and family research. *Journal of Marriage and the Family, 52,* 866–884.

Field, P. A., & Morse, J. M. (1985). *Nursing research: The application of qualitative approaches.* Rockville, MD: Aspen.

Field, T., Alpert, B., Vega-Lahr, N., Goldstein, S., & Perry, S. (1988). Hospitalization stress in children: Sensitizer and repressor coping styles. *Health Psychology, 7,* 433–445.

Field, T. M., McCabe, P. M., & Schneiderman, N. (Eds.). (1988). *Stress and coping across development.* Hillsdale, NJ: Erlbaum.

Fielding, N. G., & Lee, R. M. (1991). *Using computers in qualitative research.* Newbury Park, CA: Sage.

Fine, S. (1978). Floorplans and cartoon strips: Diagnostic techniques in working with children. *Child Psychiatry and Human Development, 9,* 33–39.

Fisher, L. (1982). Transactional theories but individual assessment: A frequent discrepancy in family research. *Family Process, 21,* 313–320.

Fisher, L., Kokes, R. F., Ransom, D. C., Phillips, S., & Rudd, P. (1985). Alternative strategies for creating "relational" family data. *Family Process, 24,* 213–224.

Folger, J. P., Hewes, D., & Poole, M. S. (1984). Coding social interaction. In B. Dervin & M. Voight (Eds.), *Progress in the communication sciences* (pp. 115–161). New York: Ablex.

Folkman, S. (1979). An analysis of coping in an adequately functioning middle-aged community sample. *Dissertation Abstracts International, 41–01,* 406B. (University Microfilms No. DDJ80–14679)

Folkman, S., & Lazarus, R. S. (1980). An analysis of coping in a middle-aged community sample. *Journal of Health and Social Behavior, 21,* 219–239.

Folkman, S., & Lazarus, R. S. (1985). *Ways of Coping.* Unpublished test. University of California at Berkeley, Berkeley, CA.

Foorman, B. R. (1974, February). *A look at reading diary studies: The state of the art and implications from cognitive–developmental theory.* Paper presented at the Special Invitational Interdisciplinary Seminar on Piagetian Theory and Its Implications for the Helping Professions, Los Angeles, CA.

Ford, D. R., & Herrick, J. (1974). Family rules: Family life styles. *American Journal of Orthopsychiatry, 44,* 61–69.

Fowlkes, M. (1980). *Behind every successful man.* New York: Columbia University Press.

Friedman, E. H. (1982). Stress and intensive care nursing: A ten-year reappraisal. *Heart–Lung, 11,* 26–28.

Friedman, M., & Rosenman, R. H. (1974). *Type A behavior and your heart.* New York: Knopf.

Friedman, M. M. (1992). *Family nursing theory and practice* (3rd ed.). Norwalk, CT: Appleton & Lange.

Furman, E. (1983). Studies in childhood bereavement. *Canadian Journal of Psychiatry, 28,* 241–247.

Furth, G. (1988). *The secret world of drawing: Healing through art.* Boston: Sego.

Gallant, M. J., & Kleinman, S. (1983). Symbolic interactionism versus ethnomethodology. *Symbolic Interaction, 6,* 1–18.

Garmezy, N. (1991). Resilience in children's adaptation to negative life events and stressed environments. *Pediatric Annals, 20,* 459–466.

Garmezy, N., & Rutter, M. (Eds.). (1983). *Stress, coping, and development in children.* New York: McGraw-Hill.

Garrod, A. C., Beal, C. R., & Shin, P. (1990). The development of moral orientation in elementary school children. *Sex-Roles, 22,* 13–27.

Garvin, B. J., Kennedy, C. W., & Cissna, K. N. (1987). Reliability in category coding systems. *Nursing Research, 37,* 52–56.

George, L. (1980). *Role transitions in later life.* Belmont, CA: Brooks/Cole.

Gilbert, L. A. (1976). Situational factors and the relationship between locus of control and psychological adjustment. *Journal of Counselling Psychology, 23,* 302–309.

Gilliss, C. L. (1983). The family as a unit of analysis: Strategies for the nurse researcher. *Advances in Nursing Science, 5,* 50–59.

Gilliss, C. L., Highley, B. L., Roberts, B. M., & Martinson, I. M. (Eds.). (1989). *Toward a science of family nursing.* Menlo Park, CA: Addison-Wesley.

Girdano, D., & Everly, G. S. (1979). *Controlling stress and tension: A holistic approach.* Englewood Cliffs, NJ: Prentice-Hall.

Gochman, D. S. (1985). Family determinants of children's concept of health and illness. In D. C. Turk & R. D. Kerns (Eds.), *Health, illness and families* (pp. 23–49). New York: Wiley.

Godwin, D. D. (1985). Simultaneous equations methods in family research. *Journal of Marriage and the Family, 47,* 9–23.

Goldsmith, H. H., Buss, A. H., Plomin, R., Rothbart, M. K., Thomas, A., Chess, S., Hinde, R. A., & McCall, R. B. (1987). Roundtable: What is temperament? Four approaches. *Child Development, 58,* 505–529.

Gollin, E. S., & Sharps, M. J. (1987). Visual perspective-taking in young children: Reduction of egocentric errors by induction of strategy. *Bulletin of the Psychonomic Society, 25,* 435–437.

Gottschalk, A. (1983). Vulnerability to stress. *American Journal of Psychotherapy, 37,* 5–23.

Grey, M., Cameron, M. E., & Thurber, F. W. (1991). Coping and adaptation in children with diabetes. *Nursing Research, 40,* 144–149.

Grobe, M. E., Ilstrup, D., & Ahmann, D. (1981). Skills needed by family members to maintain the care of an advanced cancer patient. *Cancer Nursing, 4,* 371–375.

Grotevant, H. D., & Carlson, C. I. (1987). Family interaction coding systems: A descriptive review. *Family Process, 26,* 49–76.

Guba, E. G. (1981). Criteria for assessing the trustworthiness of naturalistic inquiries. *Educational Communication and Technology Journal, 29,* 75–91.

Haggerty, R. J. (1980). Life stress, illness, and social supports. *Developmental Medicine and Child Neurology, 22,* 391–400.

Haight, G. S. (1942). Introduction. In H. D. Thoreau, *Walden* (pp. i–x). Roslyn, NY: Walter J. Black.

Haley, J. (1972). Critical overview of the present status of family interaction research. In J. Framo (Ed.), *Family Interaction.* New York: Springer.

Handel, G. (1985). Central issues in the construction of sibling relationships. In G. Handel (Ed.), *The psychosocial interior of the family* (pp. 367–394). New York: Aldine.

Hanson, C. L., Klesges, R. C., Eck, L. H., Cigrang, J. A., & Carle, D. L. (1990). Family relations, coping styles, stress, and cardiovascular disease risk factors among children and their parents. *Family Systems Medicine, 8,* 387–400.

Hanson, S. L., & Pichert, J. W. (1986). Stress and diabetes control in adolescents. *Health Psychology, 5,* 439–452.

Hargreaves, D. J. (1978). Psychological studies of children's drawings. *Educational Review, 30,* 247–254.

Hartman, R. K. (1972). An investigation of the incremental validity of human figure drawings in the diagnosis of learning disabilities. *Journal of School Psychology, 10,* 9–16.

Havighurst, R. J. (1972). *Developmental tasks and education.* New York: McKay.

Hendricks, G., & Wills, R. (1975). *The centering book.* Englewood, Cliffs, NJ: Prentice-Hall.

Hetherington, E. J. (1984). Stress and coping in children and families. *New Directions for Child Development, 24,* 7–33.

Hill, R. (1949). *Families under stress.* New York: Harper & Row.

Hill, R. (1958). Generic features of families under stress. *Social Casework, 49,* 139–150.

Hill, R. (1966). Contemporary developments in family theory. *Journal of Marriage and the Family, 28,* 10–26.

Hill, R., & Hansen, D. A. (1960). The identification of conceptual frameworks utilized in family study. *Marriage and Family Living, 22,* 299–311.

Holaday, B. (1989). The family with a chronically ill child: An interactional perspective. In C. L. Gillis, B. L. Highley, B. M. Roberts, & I. M. Martinson (Eds.), *Toward a science of family nursing* (pp. 300–321). Menlo Park, CA: Addison-Wesley.

Holaday, B., Turner-Henson, A., & Swan, J. (1991). Stability of school-age children's survey responses. *Image: Journal of Nursing Scholarship, 23,* 109–114.

Holahan, C., & Moos, R. (1985). Life stress and health: Personality, coping, and family support in stress resistance. *Journal of Personality and Social Psychology, 49,* 739–747.

Holman, T. B., & Burr, W. R. (1980). Beyond the beyond: The growth of family theories in the 1970's. *Journal of Marriage and the Family, 42,* 729–741.

Holmes, T. H., & Rahe, R. H. (1967). The social readjustment rating scale. *Journal of Psychosomatic Research, 11,* 213–218.

Holroyd, J. (1974). The questionnaire on resources and stress: An instrument to measure family response to a handicapped family member. *Journal of Community Psychology, 2,* 92–94.

Holroyd, J., & Guthrie, D. (1986). Family stress with chronic childhood illness: Cystic fibrosis, neuromuscular disease, and renal disease. *Journal of Clinical Psychology, 42,* 552–561.

Holt, R. R. (1982). Occupational stress. In L. Goldberger & S. Breznitz (Eds.), *Handbook of stress: Theoretical and clinical aspects* (pp. 419–444). New York: Macmillan.

Homans, G. C. (1958). Social behavior as exchange. *American Journal of Sociology, 63,* 597–606.

Howe, J. W., Burgess, A. W., & McCormack, A. (1987). Adolescent runaways and their drawings. *Arts in Psychotherapy, 14,* 35–40.

Hudgens, R. W. (1974). Personal catastrophe and depression: A consideration of the subject with respect to medically ill adolescents, and a requiem for retrospective life events studies. In B. S. Dohrenwend & B. P.

Dohrenwend (Eds.), *Stressful life events: Their nature and effect* (pp. 119–134). New York: Wiley.

Hunsberger, M., Love, B., & Byrne, C. (1984). A review of current approaches used to help children and parents cope with health care procedures. *Maternal–Child Nursing Journal, 13,* 145–165.

Hurwitz, A. (1980). Children as illustrators: A transcultural experience. *School Arts, 79,* 38–42.

Irish, D. (1964). Sibling interaction: A neglected aspect in family life research. *Social Forces, 42,* 279–288.

Jencks, B. (1979). *Your body: Biofeedback at its best.* Chicago: Nelson-Hall.

Jenson, M. D. (1983, March). *Studying intrapersonal communication through memoirs and journals.* Paper presented at the Annual Meeting of the International Conference on Culture and Communication, Philadelphia, PA.

Joffe, C. (1973). Taking young children seriously. In N. Denzin (Ed.), *Children and their caretakers.* New Brunswick, NJ: Transaction.

Johnson, B. H. (1990). Children's drawings as a projective technique. *Pediatric Nursing, 16,* 11–17.

Johnson, J. H. (1986). *Life events as stressors in childhood and adolescence.* Beverly Hills, CA: Sage.

Johnson, V. J. (1989). The contributions of children's histories, perceptions, and prior coping effectiveness to their behavioral responses to stress. *Dissertation Abstracts International, 50,* 1602-A (Order No. DA8921415).

Jones, G. R. (1983). Life history methodology. In G. Morgan (Ed.), *Beyond method: Strategies for social research* (pp. 147–159). Beverly Hills, CA: Sage.

Jones, R. M. (1985). Comparative study of the Kinetic Family Drawing and the Animal Kinetic Family Drawing in regard to self-concept assessment in children of divorced and intact families. *Arts in Psychotherapy, 12,* 187–196.

Jones, S. L. (1987). Psychosocial problems and the family: An overview. In M. Leahey & L. M. Wright (Eds.), *Families and psychosocial problems* (pp. 2–16). Springhouse, PA: Springhouse.

Kagan, J. (1983). Stress and coping in early development. In N. Garmezy & M. Rutter (Eds.), *Stress, coping, and development in children* (pp. 191–216). New York: McGraw-Hill.

Kanner, A. D., Coyne, J. C., Schaefer, C., & Lazarus, R. S. (1981). Comparison of two modes of stress measurement: Daily hassles and uplifts versus major life events. *Journal of Behavioral Medicine, 4,* 1–39.

Kanner, A. D., Feldman, S. S., Weinberger, D. A., & Ford, M. E. (1991). Uplifts, hassles, and adaptational outcomes in early adolescents. In A. Monat & R. S. Lazarus (Eds.), *Stress and coping: An anthology* (3rd ed., pp. 158–181). New York: Columbia University Press.

Kanner, A. D., Harrison, A., & Wertlieb, D. (1985, August). *Development of the children's hassles and uplifts scales.* Poster session presentation at the meeting of the American Psychological Association, Los Angeles, CA.

Kaplan, A. (1964). *The conduct of inquiry: Methodology for behavioral science.* San Francisco: Chandler.

Kasl, S. V., & Cooper, C. L. (Eds.). (1987). *Stress and health: Issues in research methodology.* Chichester, UK: Wiley.

Kazak, A., & Marvin, R. (1984). Differences, difficulties and adaptation: Stress and social networks in families with a handicapped child. *Family Relations, 33,* 67–77.

Kessler, R. C., & McLeod, J. D. (1984). Sex differences in vulnerability to undesirable life events. *American Sociological Review, 49,* 620–631.

Kiepenheuer, K. (1980). Spontaneous drawings of a leukemic child. *Psychosomatische Medizin, 9,* 28–38.

Kilmann, P. R., Laval, R., & Wanlass, R. L. (1978). Locus of control and perceived adjustment to life events. *Journal of Clinical Psychology, 34,* 512–513.

Kirgis, C. A., Woolsey, D. B., & Sullivan, J. J. (1977). Predicting infant Apgar scores. *Nursing Research, 26,* 439–442.

Klein, D. M. (1983). Family problem solving and family stress. In H. I. McCubbin, M. B. Sussman, & J. M. Patterson (Eds.), *Social stress and the family* (pp. 85–111). New York: Haworth.

Klein, D. M., & Jurich, J. A. (in press). Metatheory and family studies. In P. Boss, W. Doherty, R. LaRossa, W. Schumm, & S. Steinmetz (Eds.), *Sourcebook of family theories and methods: A contextual approach* New York: Plenum Press.

Knafl, K. A., & Grace, H. K. (1978). *Families across the life cycle: Studies for nursing.* Boston: Little, Brown.

Knoff, H. M., & Prout, H. T. (1985). The kinetic drawing system: A review and integration of the kinetic family and school drawing techniques. *Psychology in the Schools, 22,* 50–59.

Knudson-Cooper, M. S., & Leuchtag, A. K. (1982). The stress of a family move as a precipitating factor in children's burn accidents. *Journal of Human Stress, 8,* 32–38.

Knutson, A. S. (1991). *Parental perceptions of child stress experiences: An exploratory investigation.* Unpublished master's thesis, Brigham Young University, Provo, UT.

Kobasa, S. (1979). Stressful life events, personality, and health: An inquiry into hardiness. *Journal of Personality and Social Psychology, 37,* 1–11.

Kobasa, S. (1982). The hardy personality: Toward a social psychology of stress and health. In J. Suls & G. Sanders (Eds.), *Social psychology of health and illness* (pp. 3–32). Hindsdale, NJ: Erlbaum.

Kobasa, S., Maddi, S., & Courington, S. (1981). Personality and constitution as mediators in the stress–illness relationship. *Journal of Health and Social Behavior, 22,* 368–378.

Kobasa, S., Maddi, S., & Kahn, S. (1982). Hardiness and health: A prospective study. *Journal of Personality and Social Psychology, 42,* 168–177.

Kohlberg, L. (1964). Development of moral character and moral ideology. In L. W. Hoffman & M. L. Hoffman (Eds.), *Review of child development research* (Vol. 1, pp. 383–431). New York: Russell Sage Foundation.

Kohlberg, L. (1968). Moral development. In D. L. Sills (Ed.), *International encyclopedia of the social sciences* (pp. 404–409). New York: Macmillan.

Koop, P. M., & Keating, N. C. (1990, November). *Family stress theory: Analysis of selected models and a proposed revision.* Paper presented at the preconference workshop of the National Council on Family Relations, Seattle, WA.

Koos, E. L. (1946). *Families in trouble.* New York: Kings Crown.

Koppitz, E. M. (1983). Projective drawing with children and adolescents. *School Psychology Review, 12,* 421–427.

Krahn, G. L. (1985). The use of projective assessment techniques in pediatric settings. *Journal of Pediatric Psychology, 10,* 179–193.

Kramer, E. (1971). *Art as therapy with children.* New York: Schocken.

Krippendorf, K. (1980). *Content analysis.* Newbury Park, CA: Sage.

Kubler-Ross, E. (1981). *Living with death and dying.* New York: Macmillan.

Kuhlman, T. L., & Bieliauskas, V. J. (1976). A comparison of black and white adolescents on the HTP. *Journal of Clinical Psychology, 32,* 728–731.

Kyrios, M., & Prior, M. (1990). Temperament, stress, and family factors in behavioral adjustment of 3–5-year-old children. *International Journal of Behavioral Development, 13,* 67–93.

LaMontagne, L. L. (1984). Children's locus of control beliefs as predictors of preoperative coping behaviors. *Nursing Research, 33,* 76–79, 85.

LaMontagne, L. L. (1987). Children's preoperative coping: Replication and extension. *Nursing Research, 36,* 163–167.

LaMontagne, L. L., Mason, K. R., & Hepworth, J. T. (1985). Effects of relaxation on anxiety in children: Implications for coping with stress. *Nursing Research, 34,* 289–292.

Landgarten, H. B. (1987). *Family art psychotherapy.* New York: Brunner-Mazel.

Langer, E. (1975). The illusion of control. *Journal of Personality and Social Psychology, 32,* 311–328.

Larsen, A., & Olson, D. H. (1990). Capturing the complexity of family systems: Integrating family theory, family scores, and family analysis. In T. W. Draper & A. C. Marcos (Eds.), *Family variables* (pp. 19–47). Newbury Park, CA: Sage.

Larson, L. E. (1974). System and subsystem perception of family roles. *Journal of Marriage and the Family, 36,* 123–138.

Larzelere, R. E., & Klein, D. M. (1987). Methodology. In M. B. Sussman & S. K. Steinmetz (Eds.), *Handbook of marriage and the family* (pp. 125–155). New York: Plenum Press.

Lasky, P., Buckwalter, K. C., Whall, A., Lederman, R., Speer, J., McLane, A., King, J. M., & White, M. A. (1985). Developing an instrument for the assessment of family dynamics. *Western Journal of Nursing Research, 7,* 40–57.

Lavee, Y., & Dollahite, D. C. (1991). The linkage between theory and research in family science. *Journal of Marriage and the Family, 53,* 361–373.

Lavee, Y., & Olson, D. H. (1991). Family types and response to stress. *Journal of Marriage and the Family, 53,* 786–798.

Lazarus, R. S. (1966). *Psychological stress and the coping process.* New York: McGraw-Hill.

Lazarus, R. S. (1981). The stress and coping paradigm. In C. Esdorfer, D. Cohen, A. Kleinman, & P. Maxim (Eds.), *Models for clinical psychopathology* (pp. 177–214). New York: Spectrum.

Lazarus, R. S. (1982). Thoughts on the relations between emotion and cognition. *American Psychologist, 37,* 1019–1042.

Lazarus, R. S. (1984). On the primacy of cognition. *American Psychologist, 39,* 124–219.

Lazarus, R. S., & Folkman, S. (1984). *Stress, appraisal, and coping.* New York: Springer.

Lazarus, R. S., & Launier, R. (1978). Stress-related transactions between person and environment. In L. A. Pervin & M. Lewis (Eds.), *Perspectives in interactional psychology* (pp. 287–327) New York: Plenum Press.

Lee, H. J. (1983). Analysis of a concept: Hardiness. *Oncology Forum, 10,* 32–35.

Leonard, B. J. (1991). Siblings of chronically ill children: A question of vulnerability versus resilience. *Pediatric Annals, 20,* 501–506.

Levenberg, S. B. (1975). Professional training, psychodiagnostic skill, and kinetic family drawings. *Journal of Personality Assessment, 39,* 389–393.

Levinger, G. (1977). Re-viewing the close relationship. In G. Levinger & H. L. Raush (Eds.), *Close relationships.* Amherst, MA: University of Massachusetts Press.

Levinson, R. M., & Ramsey, G. (1979). Dangerousness, stress, and mental health evaluations. *Journal of Health and Social Behavior, 20,* 178–187.

Levy, S. M. (Ed.). (1982). *Biological mediators of behavior and disease: Neoplasia.* New York: Elsevier Biomedical.

Lewis, C. E., Siegel, J. M., & Lewis, M. A. (1984). Feeling bad: Exploring sources of distress among preadolescent children. *American Journal of Public Health, 74,* 117–122.

Linville, P. (1987). Self-complexity as a cognitive buffer against stress-related illness and depression. *Journal of Personality and Social Psychology, 52,* 663–676.

Litman, T. J. (1974). The family as a basic unit in health and medical care: A social behavioral overview. *Social Science and Medicine, 8,* 495–519.

Litman, T., & Venters, M. (1979). Research on healthcare and the family: A methodological overview. *Social Science Medicine, 13A,* 379–385.

Long, E. C. (1990). Measuring dyadic perspective-taking: Two scales for assessing perspective-taking in marriage and similar dyads. *Education and Psychological Measurement, 50,* 91–103.

Lowenfeld, V., & Brittain, W. L. (1975). *Creative and mental growth.* New York: Macmillan.

Lowman, J. (1980). Measurement of family affective structure. *Journal of Personality Assessment, 44,* 130–141.

Lucio del Raggi, E., & Huazo, V. M. C. (1984). Imagen corporal en el niño urémico [Body image in the uremic child]. *Salud Mental, 7,* 9–14.

Lumley, M. A., Abeles, L. A., Melamed, B. G., Pistone, L. M., & Johnson,

J. H. (1990). Coping outcomes in children undergoing stressful medical procedures: The role of child–environment variables. *Behavioral Assessment, 12,* 223–238.

Malchiodi, C. A. (1990). *Breaking the silence: Art therapy with children from violent homes.* New York: Brunner/Mazel.

Manning, M., Manning, G., & Hughes, J. (1987). Journals in first grade: What children write. *Reading Teacher, 41,* 311–315.

Manning, T. M. (1987). Aggression depicted in abused children's drawings. *Arts in Psychotherapy, 14,* 15–24.

Martin, R., & Lefcourt, H. (1983). Sense of humor as a moderator of the relationship between stressors and moods. *Journal of Personality and Social Psychology, 45,* 1313–1324.

Martin, R. P. (1983). Projective procedures: An ethical dilemma. *Psychological Abstracts, 71,* 19424.

Mason, J. W. (1975). A historical view of the stress field. Part II. *Journal of Human Stress, 1,* 22–36.

Masten, A. S. (1985). Stress, coping, and children's health. *Pediatric Annals, 14,* 543–547.

Masuda, M., Culter, D. L., Hein, L., & Holmes, T. H. (1978). Life events and prisoners. *Archives of General Psychiatry, 35,* 197–203.

Matheny, K. B., & Cupp, P. (1983). Control, desirability, and anticipation as moderating variables between life change and illness. *Journal of Human Stress, 9,* 14–23.

Matteson, M. T., & Ivancevich, J. M. (1982). Type A and B behavior patterns and self-reported health symptoms and stress: Examining individual and organizational fit. *Journal of Occupational Medicine, 24,* 585–589.

Maurin, J. (1983). A symbolic interaction perspective of the family. In I. W. Clements & F. B. Roberts (Eds.), *Family health: A theoretical approach to nursing care.* New York: Wiley.

McCranie, E., Lambert, V., & Lambert, C. (1987). Work stress, hardiness, and burnout among hospital staff nurses. *Nursing Research, 36,* 374–378.

McCubbin, H. I., Comeau, J., & Harkins, J. (1979). *Family inventory for management (FIRM).* St. Paul: University of Minnesota.

McCubbin, H. I., & Figley, C. R. (1983). *Stress and the family: Coping with normative transitions* (Vol. 1). New York: Brunner/Mazel.

McCubbin, H. I., Joy, C. B., Cauble, A. E., Comeau, J. K., Patterson, J. M., & Needle, R. H. (1980). Family stress and coping: A decade review. *Journal of Marriage and the Family, 42,* 855–871.

McCubbin, H. I., Larsen, A. S., & Olson, D. H. (1982). *F-COPES: Family coping strategies.* St. Paul, MN: University of Minnesota.

McCubbin, H. I., & McCubbin, M. A. (1988). Typologies of resilient families: Emerging roles of social class and ethnicity. *Family Relations, 37,* 247–254.

McCubbin, H. I., McCubbin, M. A., Cauble, A., & Nevin, R. (1979). *Coping health inventory for parents (CHIP).* St. Paul, MN: University of Minnesota.

McCubbin, H. I., & Patterson, J. (1983). The family stress process: The double ABCX model of adjustment and adaptation. In H. I. McCubbin, M. Sussman, & J. Patterson (Eds.), *Social stress and the family: Advances in developments in family stress theory and research* (pp. 7-37). New York: Haworth.

McCubbin, H. I., Patterson, J., & Wilson, L. (1983). *Family inventory of life events and changes (FILE): Research instrument.* St. Paul, MN: University of Minnesota.

McCubbin, H. I., Sussman, M., & Patterson, J. (Eds.). (1983). *Social stress and the family: Advances in developments in family stress theory and research.* New York: Haworth.

McCubbin, M. A. (1989). Family stress and family strengths: A comparison of single- and two-parent families with handicapped children. *Research in Nursing and Health, 12,* 101-110.

McCubbin, M. A., & McCubbin, H. I. (1987). Family stress theory and assessment: The *t*-Double ABCX model of family adjustment and adaptation. In H. I. McCubbin & A. Thompson (Eds.), *Family assessment inventories for research and practice* (pp. 3-32). Madison, WI: University of Wisconsin.

McCubbin, M. A., & McCubbin, H. I. (in press). Family coping with illness: The resiliency model of family stress, adjustment, and adaptation. In C. Danielson, B. Hamel-Bissell, & P. Winstead-Fry (Eds.), *Families, health, and illness.* St. Louis, MO: Mosby.

McCubbin, M. A., McCubbin, H. I., & Thompson, A. I. (1986). *Family hardiness index.* Madison, WI: University of Wisconsin.

McCubbin, M. A., McCubbin, H. I., & Thompson, A. I. (1988). *Family problem solving communication.* Madison, WI: University of Wisconsin.

McKay, M., Davis, M., & Fanning, P. (1981). *Thoughts and feelings: The art of cognitive stress intervention.* Richmond, CA: New Harbinger.

McNamee, A. (Ed.). (1982). *Children and stress: Helping children cope.* Washington, DC: Association for Childhood Education International.

McNiff, K. (1982). Sex difference in children's art. *Journal of Education, 164,* 271-289.

Mechanic, D. (1983). Adolescent health and illness behavior: Review of literature and a new hypothesis for the study of stress. *Journal of Human Stress, 9,* 4-13.

Mederer, H., & Hill, R. (1983). Critical transitions over the family life span: Theory and research. In H. I. McCubbin, M. B. Sussman, & J. M. Patterson (Eds.), *Social stress and the family.* New York: Haworth.

Menaghan, E. G. (1983). Individual coping efforts and family studies: Conceptual and methodological issues. In H. I. McCubbin, M. B. Sussman, & J. M. Patterson (Eds.), *Social stress and the family.* New York: Haworth.

Meng, A., & Zastowny, G. (1982). Preparation for hospitalization: A stress inoculation training program for parents and children. *Maternal-Child Nursing Journal, 11,* 87-94.

Mercer, R. (1989). Theoretical perspective on the family. In C. L. Gilliss, B. L. Highley, B. M. Roberts, & I. M. Martinson (Eds.), *Toward a science of family nursing* (pp. 9–36). Menlo Park, CA: Addison-Wesley.

Meyer, R. J., & Haggerty, R. J. (1962). Streptococcal infection in families: Factors affecting individual susceptibility. *Pediatrics, 29,* 539–549.

Miljkovitch, M. (1984–1985). Les dessins de maisons d'une enfant entre 4½ et 10 ans [Drawings of houses made by a child between the ages of 4½ and 10 years]. *Bulletin de Psychologie, 38,* 199–215.

Miljkovitch, M., & Irvine, G. M. (1982). Comparison of drawing performances of schizophrenics, other psychiatric patients and normal schoolchildren on Draw-A-Village task. *Arts in Psychotherapy, 9,* 203–216.

Miller, B. C., & Sollie, D. L. (1980). Normal stresses during the transition to parenthood. *Family Relations, 29,* 29–35.

Miller, M. J., Tobacyk, J. M., & Wilcox, C. T. (1985). Daily hassles and uplifts as perceived by adolescents. *Psychological Reports, 56,* 221–222.

Miller, M. J., Wilcox, C. T., & Soper, B. (1985). Measuring hassles and uplifts among adolescents: A different approach to the study of stress. *School Counselor, 33,* 107–110.

Miller, T. W. (1981). Life events scaling: Clinical methodological issues. *Nursing Research, 30,* 316–320A.

Monat, A., & Lazarus, R. S. (Eds.). (1991). *Stress and coping: An anthology* (3rd ed.). New York: Columbia University Press.

Monroe, S. M. (1983). Major and minor life events as predictors of psychological distress: Further issues and findings. *Journal of Behavioral Medicine, 6,* 189–205.

Moos, R. H. (1974). Determinants of physiological responses to symbolic stimuli: The role of the social environment. *International Journal of Psychiatry in Medicine, 5,* 389–399.

Moos, R. H., Cronkite, R. C., Billings, A. G., & Finney, J. W. (1984). *Health and daily living form manual.* Palo Alto, CA: Stanford University Press.

Morrison, B. (1974). The importance of a balanced system. *Man–environment systems, 4,* 171–178.

Mostkoff, D. L., & Lazarus, P. J. (1983). The kinetic family drawing: The reliability of an objective scoring system. *Psychology in the Schools, 20,* 16–20.

Mullan, J. T. (1983, October). *The (mis)meaning of life events in family stress theory and research.* Paper presented at the Preconference Theory Construction and Research Methodology Workshop, National Council on Family Relations Annual Meeting, St. Paul, MN.

Murphy, L. B. (1974). Coping, vulnerability, and resilience in childhood. In G. V. Coelho, D. A. Hamburg, & J. E. Adams (Eds.), *Coping and adaptation* (pp. 69–100). New York: Basic.

Murphy, L. B., & Moriarty, A. E. (1976). *Vulnerability, coping, and growth: From infancy to adolescence.* New Haven, CT: Yale University Press.

Nathan, S. (1973). Body image in chronically obese children as reflected in figure drawings. *Journal of Personality Assessment, 37,* 456–463.

Norbeck, J. (1981). Social support: A model for clinical research and application. *Advances in Nursing Science, 3,* 43–59.

Nuckolls, K. B., Cassel, J., & Kaplan, B. H. (1972). Psychosocial assets, life crisis, and the prognosis of pregnancy. *American Journal of Epidemiology, 95,* 431–444.

Oliveri, M. E., & Reiss, D. (1982). Families' schemata of social relationships. *Family Process, 21,* 295–311.

Olson, D. H. (1977). Insiders' and outsiders' views of relationships: Research studies. In G. Levinger & H. L. Raush (Eds.), *Close relationships: Perspectives on the meaning of intimacy* (pp. 115–135). Amherst, MA: University of Massachusetts Press.

Olson, D. H. (1985). Commentary: Struggling with congruence across theoretical models and methods. *Family Process, 24,* 203–211.

Olson, D. H., McCubbin, H. I., Barnes, H., Larsen, A., Muxen, M., & Wilson, M. (1983). *Families: What makes them work.* Beverly Hills, CA: Sage.

Olson, D., McCubbin, H., Barnes, H., Larsen, A., Muxen, M., & Wilson, M. (Eds.). (1984). *Family inventories.* St. Paul, MN: University of Minnesota.

Olson, D. H., Sprenkle, D. H., & Russell, C. S. (1979). Circumplex model of marital and family systems: I. Cohesion and adaptability dimensions, family types, and clinical application. *Family Process, 8,* 3–28.

O'Neill, C., & Sorensen, E. S. (1991). Home care of the elderly: A family perspective. *Advances in Nursing Science, 13,* 18–37.

Padilla, E. R., Rohsenow, D. J., & Bergman, A. B. (1976). Predicting accident frequency in children. *Pediatrics, 58,* 223–226.

Panzarine, S. (1985). Coping: Conceptual and methodological issues. *Advances in Nursing Science, 7,* 49–57.

Parkes, K. R. (1984). Locus of control, cognitive appraisal, and coping in stressful episodes. *Journal of Personality and Social Psychology, 46,* 655–668.

Paterson, J. G., & Janzen, H. L. (1984). Another reply to Martin—Projective procedures: An ethical dilemma. *School Psychologist, 38,* 8–9.

Patterson, J. M. (1991). Family resilience to the challenge of a child's disability. *Pediatric Annals, 20,* 491–499.

Paykel, E. S. (1974). Life stress and psychiatric disorder: Applications of the clinical approach. In B. S. Dohrenwend & B. P. Dohrenwend (Eds.), *Stressful life events: Their nature and effects* (pp. 135–149). New York: Wiley.

Pearlin, L. I. (1991). Life strains and psychological distress among adults. In A. Monat & R. S. Lazarus (Eds.), *Stress and coping: An anthology* (3rd ed., pp. 319–336). New York: Columbia University Press.

Pearlin, L. I., & Lieberman, M. A. (1979). Social sources of emotional distress. In R. G. Simmons (Ed.), *Research in community mental health.* Greenwich, CT: JAI Press.

Pearlin, L., & Schooler, C. (1978). The structure of coping. *Journal of Health and Social Behavior, 19,* 2–21.

Peck, M. S. (1978). *The road less traveled.* New York: Simon & Schuster.

Peterson, L. (1989). Coping by children undergoing stressful medical procedures: Some conceptual, methodological, and therapeutic issues. *Journal of Consulting and Clinical Psychology, 57,* 380–387.

Piaget, J. (1952). *The origins of intelligence in children.* New York: International Universities Press.

Pidgeon, V. (1981). Functions of preschool children's questions in coping with hospitalization. *Research in Nursing and Health, 4,* 229–235.

Pless, J. B., & Satterwhite, B. (1973). A measure of family function and its application. *Social Science and Medicine, 7,* 613–621.

Pollock, S. E. (1986). Human responses to chronic illness: Physiologic and psychosocial adaptation. *Nursing Research, 35,* 90–95.

Pollock, S. E. (1989). Adaptive responses to diabetes mellitus. *Western Journal of Nursing Research, 11,* 265–280.

Poster, E. C. (1983). Stress immunization: Techniques to help children cope with hospitalization. *Maternal–Child Nursing Journal, 12,* 119–134.

Powell, T. H., & Ogle, P. A. (1985). *Brothers and sisters: A special part of exceptional families.* Baltimore: Paul H. Brookes.

Price, J. H. (1985). A model for explaining adolescent stress. *Health Education, 16,* 36–40.

Prytula, R. E., & Thompson, N. D. (1973). Analysis of emotional indicators in human figure drawings as related to self-esteem. *Perceptual Motor Skills, 37,* 456–463.

Rahe, R. H., McKean, J. D., & Arthur, R. J. (1972). A longitudinal study of life change and illness patterns I. *Psychosomatic Research, 10,* 355–366.

Rakowski, W., Julius, M., Hickey, T., Verbrugge, L. M., & Halter, J. B. (1988). Daily symptoms and behavioral responses. *Medical Care, 26,* 278–297.

Ransom, D. C., Fisher, L., Phillips, S., Kokes, R. F., & Weiss, R. (1990). The logic of measurement in family research. In T. W. Draper & A. C. Marcos (Eds.), *Family variables* (pp. 48–63). Newbury Park, CA: Sage.

Reason, P., & Rowan, J. (Eds.). (1981). *Human inquiry: A sourcebook of a new paradigm for research.* New York: Wiley.

Reiss, D. (1981). *The family's construction of reality.* Cambridge, MA: Harvard University Press.

Richardson, G. E., Beall, S., & Jessup, G. T. (1983). The efficacy of a three-week stress management unit for high school students. *Health Education, 14,* 12–15.

Riordan, R. J., & Verdel, A. C. (1991). Evidence of sexual abuse in children's art products. *School Counselor, 39,* 116–121.

Riskin, J., & Faunce, E. (1972). An evaluative overview of family interaction research. *Family Process, 11,* 365–456.

Robins, L. N. (1983). Some methodological problems and research directions in the study of the effects of stress on children. In N. Garmezy & M. Rutter (Eds.), *Stress, coping, and development in children* (pp. 335–346). New York: McGraw-Hill.

Robbins, P. R., & Tanck, R. H. (1982). Further research using a psychological diary technique to investigate psychosomatic relationships. *Journal of Clinical Psychology, 38,* 356–359.

Roberts, C. S., & Feetham, S. L. (1982). Assessing family functioning across three areas of relationships. *Nursing Research, 31,* 231–235.

Roberts, F. B. (1983). Infant behavior and the transition to parenthood. *Nursing Research, 32,* 213–217.

Roberts, J. G., Browne, G., Streiner, D., Byrne, C., Brown, B., & Love, B. (1987). Analyses of coping responses and adjustment: Stability of conclusions. *Nursing Research, 36,* 94–97.

Roche, M. (1973). *Phenomenology, language, and the social sciences.* Boston: Routledge & Paul.

Rodgers, R. H. (1964). Toward a theory of family development. *Journal of Marriage and the Family, 26,* 262–270.

Rogers, M. E. (1983). Science of unitary human beings: A paradigm for nursing. In I. W. Clements & F. B. Roberts (Eds.), *Family health: A theoretical approach to nursing care* (pp. 219–228). New York: Wiley.

Roghmann, K. J., & Haggerty, R. J. (1972). Family stress and the use of health services. *International Journal of Epidemiology, 1,* 279–286.

Roth, D., & Holmes, D. (1985). Influence of physical fitness in determining the impact of stressful life events on physical and psychological health. *Psychosomatic Medicine, 47,* 164–173.

Rothbaum, F., Wolfer, J., & Visintainer, M. (1979). Coping behavior and locus of control in children. *Journal of Personality, 47,* 118–135.

Rotter, J. B. (1966). Generalized expectancies for internal versus external control of reinforcement. *Psychological Monographs, 80*(1, Whole No. 609).

Rubin, J. A. (1984). *Child art therapy: Understanding and helping children grow through art* (2nd ed.). New York: Van Nostrand Reinhold.

Ruddick, S. (1982). Maternal thinking. In B. Thorne & M. Yalom (Eds.), *Rethinking the family* (pp. 213–230). New York: Longman.

Rutter, M. (1982). Temperament: Concepts, issues, and problems. *Ciba Foundation Symposium, 89,* 1–19.

Rutter, M. (1983). Stress, coping, and development: Some issues and some questions. In N. Garmezy & M. Rutter (Eds.), *Stress, coping, and development in children* (pp. 1–41). New York: McGraw-Hill.

Rutter, M. (1987). Temperament, personality, and personality disorder. *British Journal of Psychiatry, 150,* 443–458.

Ryan, N. M. (1988). The stress–coping process in school-age children: Gaps in the knowledge needed for health promotion. *Advances in Nursing Science, 11,* 1–12.

Ryan, N. M. (1989). Stress-coping strategies identified from school age children's perspective. *Research in Nursing and Health, 12,* 111–122.

Ryan-Wenger, N. M. (1990). Development and psychometric properties of the schoolagers' coping strategies inventory. *Nursing Research, 39,* 344–349.

Sandelowski, M. (1986). The problem of rigor in qualitative research. *Advances in Nursing Science, 8,* 27–37.

Sandler, I. N., & Block, M. (1979). Life stress and maladaptation of children. *American Journal of Community Psychology, 7,* 425–440.

Saunders, A., & Remsberg, B. (1984). *The stress-proof child: A loving parent's guide.* New York: Holt, Rinehart & Winston.

Savedra, M., & Tesler, M. (1981). Coping strategies of hospitalized school-age children. *Western Journal of Nursing Research, 3,* 371–384.

Schatzman, L., & Strauss, A. (1973). *Field research: Strategies for a natural sociology.* Englewood Cliffs, NJ: Prentice-Hall.

Scheier, M., Weintraub, J., & Carver, C. (1986). Coping with stress: Divergent strategies of optimists and pessimists. *Journal of Personality and Social Psychology, 51,* 1257–1264.

Schilling, R. G., Gilchrist, L. D., & Schinke, S. P. (1984). Coping and social support in families of developmentally disabled children. *Family Relations: Journal of Applied Family and Child Studies, 33,* 47–54.

Schilling, R., Schinke, S., & Kirkham, M. (1985). Coping with a handicapped child: Differences between mothers and fathers. *Social Science and Medicine, 21,* 857–863.

Schornstein, H. M., & Derr, J. (1978). The many applications of kinetic family drawings in child abuse. *British Journal of Projective Psychology and Personality Study, 23,* 33–35.

Schumm, W. R. (1982). Integrating theory, measurement and data analysis in family studies survey research. *Journal of Marriage and the Family, 44,* 983–999.

Schvaneveldt, J. D., & Ihinger, M. (1979). Sibling relationships in the family. In W. Burr, R. Hill, F. I. Nye, & I. L. Reiss (Eds.), *Contemporary theories about the family* (Vol. 1). New York: Free Press.

Scott, J. (1986). Gender: A useful category of historical analysis. *American Historical Review, 91,* 1053–1075.

Seamonds, B. C. (1982). Stress factors and their effect on absenteeism in a corporate employee group. *Journal of Occupational Medicine, 24,* 393–397.

Segal, R. M. (1984). Helping children express grief through symbolic communication. *Social Casework: The Journal of Contemporary Social Work, 65,* 590–599.

Selye, H. (1956). *The stress of life.* New York: McGraw-Hill.

Selye, H. (1974). *Stress without distress.* New York: New American Library.

Selye, H. (1983). The stress concept: Past, present, and future. In C. L. Cooper (Ed.), *Stress research: Issues for the eighties* (pp. 1–20). New York: Wiley.

Sharrer, V. W., & Ryan-Wenger, N. M. (1991). Measurements of stress and coping among school-aged children with and without recurrent abdominal pain. *Journal of School Health, 61,* 86–91.

Shaw, D. S., & Emery, R. E. (1988). Chronic family adversity and school-age children's adjustment. *Journal of the American Academy of Child Adolescent Psychiatry, 27,* 200–206.

Shenker, I. (1990). Winsome, weird and wonderful—art made by children. *Smithsonian, 21,* 148–157.

Shrewsbury, J. (1982). Painting: A coping device for preschool hospitalized children. *Maternal–Child Nursing Journal, 11,* 11–16.

Siegel, B. S. (1986). *Love, medicine, and miracles.* New York: Harper & Row.

Sinnema, G. (1991). Resilience among children with special health-care needs and among their families. *Pediatric Annals, 20,* 483–486.

Smilkstein, G. (1978). The family APGAR: A proposal for a family function test and its use by physicians. *The Journal of Family Practice, 6,* 1231–1239.

Smith, G. M. (1985). The collaborative drawing technique. *Journal of Personality Assessment, 49,* 582–585.

Sorensen, D. M. (1986, November). *What you expect is what you get: The connection between theories and outcomes in the physical and behavioral sciences.* Paper presented at Brigham Young University Spheres of Influence Conference, Provo, UT.

Sorensen, E. S. (1988). *Daily stressors and coping responses in well children.* Unpublished doctoral dissertation, University of Utah, Salt Lake City, UT.

Sorensen, E. S. (1989). Using children's diaries as a research instrument. *Journal of Pediatric Nursing, 4,* 427–431.

Sorensen, E. S. (1990). Children's coping responses. *Journal of Pediatric Nursing, 5,* 259–267.

Sorensen, E. S. (1991). Identification of stress buffers in school age children. *Journal of Community Health Nursing, 8,* 15–24.

Sorensen, E. S. (in press-a). Daily life stress in children. In J. Humphrey (Ed.), *Human stress: Current selected research* (Vol. 5). New York: AMS Press.

Sorensen, E. S. (in press-b). Daily stressors and coping responses: A comparison between rural and suburban children. *Public Health Nursing.*

Spielberger, C. D. (Ed.). (1966). *Anxiety and behavior.* New York: Academic Press.

Sprey, J. (1988). Current theorizing on the family: An appraisal. *Journal of Marriage and the Family, 50,* 875–890.

Stawar, T. L., & Stawar, D. E. (1987). Family kinetic drawings as a screening instrument. *Perceptual & Motor Skills, 65,* 810.

Steeves, H. L., & Bostian, L. R. (1982). A comparison of cooperation levels of diary and questionnaire respondents. *Journalism Quarterly, 59,* 610–616.

Steinhardt, L. (1989). *Six starting points in art therapy with children.* New York: Wiley.

Steinmetz, J. I., Kaplan, R. M., & Miller, G. L. (1982). Stress management: An assessment questionnaire for evaluating interventions and comparing groups. *Journal of Occupational Medicine, 24,* 923–931.

Stephan, P. M. (1971). *The secret of eternal youth.* New York: Arco.

Stern, P. M. (1990). The relation of cognitive development to children's coping response to marital separation. *Dissertation Abstracts International, 51,* 1558-A (Order No. DA9026094).

Stevenson-Hinde, J., & Simpson, A. E. (1982). Temperament and relationships. *Ciba Foundation Symposium, 89,* 51–65.

Straus, M. A. (1964). Measuring families. In H. T. Christensen (Ed.), *Handbook of marriage and the family.* Chicago: Rand McNally.

Sturner, R. A., Rothbaum, F., Visintainer, M., & Wolfer, J. (1980). The effects of stress on children's human figure drawings. *Journal of Clinical Psychology, 36,* 324–331.

Suls, J., & Fletcher, B. (1985). The relative efficacy of avoidant and nonavoidant coping strategies: A meta-analysis. *Health Psychology, 4,* 249–288.

Swanson-Kauffman, K. M. (1986). A combined qualitative methodology for nursing research. *Advances in Nursing Science, 8,* 58–69.

Swogger, G. (1981). Toward understanding stress: A map of the territory. *Journal of School Health, 51,* 29–33.

Tate, F. B. (1989). Symbols in the graphic art of the dying. *The Arts in Psychotherapy, 16,* 115–120.

Taylor, M. (1988). Conceptual perspective-taking: Children's ability to distinguish what they know from what they see. *Child Development, 59,* 703–718.

Taylor, S. C. (1980). The effect of chronic childhood illnesses upon well siblings. *Maternal-Child Nursing Journal, 9,* 109–116.

Taylor, S. E. (1983). Adjustment to threatening events: A theory of cognitive adaptation. *American Psychologist, 38,* 1161–1173.

Taylor, S. E., & Brown, J. D. (1988). Illusion and well-being: A social psychological perspective on mental health. *Psychological Bulletin, 103,* 193–210.

Terr, L. (1979). Children of Chowchilla. *Psychoanalytic Study of the Child, 24,* 552–623.

Tesch, R. (1987). *Qualitative data management with the personal computer.* Paper presented at the American Education Research Association Annual Meeting, Washington, DC.

Thoits, P. (1986). Social support as coping assistance. *Consulting and Clinical Psychology, 54,* 416–432.

Thomas, R. B., & Barnard, K. E. (1986, June). Understanding families: A look at measures and methodologies. *Zero to Three,* 11–14.

Tholome, E. (1984–1985). Les aspects génétiques et culturels de l'expression graphique. Etude de 2,700 dessins d'enfants et d'adultes sur le thème "Le repas familial" [Developmental and cultural factors influencing graphic expression: Study of 2,700 drawings by children and adults on the theme "the family meal"]. *Bulletin de Psychologie, 38,* 243–254.

Thomas, A., & Chess, S. (1977). *Temperament and development.* New York: Brunner-Mazel.

Thomas, R. B. (1987). Methodological problems in family health care research. *Journal of Marriage and the Family, 49,* 65–70.

Thomas, R. B., & Barnard, K. E. (1986, June). Understanding families: A look at measures and methodologies. *Zero to Three,* 11–14.

Thoresen, C. E., Eagleston, J. R., Kirmil-Gray, D., & Bracke, P. E. (1985). *Exploring the Type A behavior pattern in children and adolescents.* Paper presented at the American Psychological Association Annual Meeting, Los Angeles, CA.

Thorne, B. (1986). Girls and boys together . . . but mostly apart: Gender arrangements in elementary schools. In W. Hartup & Z. Rubin (Eds.), *Relationships and development.* Hillsdale, NJ: Erlbaum.

Touliatos, J., Perlmutter, B. F., & Straus, M. A. (Eds.). (1990). *Handbook of family measurement techniques.* Newbury Park, CA: Sage.

Uphold, C. R., & Strickland, O. L. (1989). Issues related to the unit of analysis in family nursing research. *Western Journal of Nursing Research,* 11, 405–417.

Ventura, J. N., & Stevenson, M. B. (1986). Relations of mothers' and fathers' reports of infant temperament, parents' psychological functioning, and family characteristics. *Merrill-Palmer Quarterly, 32,* 275–289.

Wadeson, H. (1980). *Art psychotherapy.* New York: Wiley.

Wagnild, G., & Young, H. M. (1991). Another look at hardiness. *Image: Journal of Nursing Scholarship, 23,* 257–259.

Waldrop, M., & Halverson, C. (1975). Intensive and extensive peer behavior: Longitudinal and cross-sectional analysis. *Child Development, 46,* 19–26.

Walker, A. J. (1985). Reconceptualizing family stress. *Journal of Marriage and the Family, 45,* 827–837.

Walker, C. L. (1986). Stress and coping in the siblings of children with cancer. *Dissertation Abstracts International, 47-07,* 2841B. (University Microfilms No. DA8624430)

Walker, C. L. (1988). Stress and coping in siblings of childhood cancer patients. *Nursing Research, 37,* 208–212.

Walker, L. J. (1980). Cognitive and perspective-taking prerequisites for moral development. *Child Development, 51,* 131–139.

Walters, L. H., Pittman, J. F., & Norrell, J. E. (1984). Development of a quantitative measure of a family from self-reports of family members. *Journal of Family Issues, 5,* 497–514.

Wannon, M. (1990). Children's control beliefs about controllable and uncontrollable events: Their relationship to stress resilience and psychosocial adjustment. *Dissertation Abstracts International, 51,* 3182-B (Order No. DA9032789).

Weinberg, S. L., & Richardson, M. S. (1981). Dimensions of stress in early parenting. *Journal of Consulting Clinical Psychology, 48,* 686–693.

Werner, H. (1948). *Comparative psychology of mental development.* New York: International Universities Press.

Werner, E. E., & Smith, R. S. (1982). *Vulnerable but invincible: A longitudinal study of resilient children and youth.* New York: McGraw-Hill.

Wertlieb, D., Weigel, C., & Feldstein, M. (1987). Measuring children's coping. *American Journal of Orthopsychiatry, 57,* 548–560.

Wethington, E., McLeod, J. D., & Kessler, R. C. (1987). The importance of life events in explaining sex differences in psychological distress. In R.

C. Barnett, L. Biener, & G. K. Baruch (Eds.), *Gender and stress* (pp. 144–156). New York: Free Press.

Whall, A. L. (1980). Congruence between existing theories of family functioning and nursing theories. *Advances in Nursing Science, 3,* 59–67.

Whall, A. L. (1981). Nursing theory and the assessment of families. *Journal of Psychiatric Nursing, 19,* 30–36.

Whall, A. L., & Fawcett, J. (1991). *Family theory development in nursing: State of the science and art.* Philadelphia: F. A. Davis.

Wheeler, R. J., & Frank, M. A. (1988, Summer). Identification of stress buffers. *Behavioral Medicine,* 778–89.

White, J. M. (1984). Not the sum of its parts. *Journal of Family Issues, 5,* 515–518.

Wiebe, D., & McCallum, D. (1986). Health practices and hardiness as mediators in the stress–illness relationship. *Health Psychology, 5,* 425–438.

Wilson, D., & Ratekin, C. (1990, March). Children's drawings as an assessment tool. *Nurse Practitioner,* 23–35.

Wiseman, J. P. (1981). The family and its researchers in the eighties: Retrenching, renewing, revitalizing. *Journal of Marriage and the Family, 43,* 263–266.

Witkin-Lanoil, G. (1984). *The female stress syndrome.* New York: Berkley.

Witkin-Lanoil, G. (1986). *The male stress syndrome.* New York: Newmarket Press.

Witmer, J., Rich, C., Barcikowski, R., & Mague, J. (1983). Psychosocial characteristics mediating the stress response: An exploratory study. *Personnel and Guidance Journal, 62,* 73–77.

Wolchick, S. A., Sandler, I. N., Braver, S. L., & Fogas, B. S. (1986). Events of parental divorce: Stressfulness ratings by children, parents, and clinicians. *American Journal of Community Psychology, 14,* 59–74.

Wolfer, J. A., & Visintainer, M. A. (1975). Pediatric surgical patients' and parents' stress responses and adjustment as a function of psychologic preparation and stress-point nursing care. *Nursing Research, 24,* 244–253.

Wolfer, J. A., & Visintainer, M. A. (1979). Prehospital psychological preparation for tonsillectomy patients: Effects on children's and parents' adjustment. *Pediatrics, 74,* 646–655.

Woods, N. F. (1987). Women's health: The menstrual cycle. Premenstrual symptoms: Another look. *Public Health Reports, 2,* 106–112.

Woolfolk, R. L., & Lehrer, P. M. (Eds.). (1984). *Principles and practice of stress management.* New York: Guilford Press.

Woolfolk, R. L., Lehrer, P. M., McCann, B. S., & Rooney, A. J. (1982). Effects of progressive relaxation and meditation on cognitive and somatic manifestations of daily stress. *Behaviour Research and Therapy, 20,* 461–467.

Wright, L. M., & Leahey, M. (Eds.). (1987). *Families and psychosocial problems.* Springhouse, PA: Springhouse.

Yamamoto, K. (1979). Children's ratings of the stressfulness of experiences. *Developmental Psychology, 15,* 581–582.

Yamamoto, K. & Byrnes, D. A. (1984). Classroom social status, ethnicity, and ratings of stressful events. *Journal of Educational Research, 77,* 283–286.

Yamamoto, K., & Felsenthal, H. M. (1982). Stressful experiences of children: Professional judgments. *Psychological Reports, 50,* 1087–1093.

Yamamoto, K., Soliman, A., Parsons, J., & Davies, O. L. (1987). Voices in unison: Stressful events in the lives of children in six countries. *Journal of Child Psychology and Psychiatry, 28,* 855–864.

Youngs, B. B. (1985). *Stress in children: How to recognize, avoid, and overcome it.* New York: Arbor House.

Zastowny, T. R., Kirschenbaum, D. S., & Meng, A. L. (1986). Coping skills training for children: Effects on distress before, during, and after hospitalization for surgery. *Health Psychology. 5,* 231–247.

Zeitlin, S. (1980). Assessing coping behavior. *American Journal of Orthopsychiatry, 50,* 139–144.

Zeitlin, S. (1985). *Coping Inventory: A measure of adaptive behavior.* Bensenville, IL: Scholastic Testing Service.

Zlatich, D., Kenny, T. J., Sila, U., & Huang, S. W. (1982). Parent–child life events: Relation to treatment in asthma. *Journal of Developmental Behavioral Pediatrics, 3,* 69–72.

Zucker, K. J., Finegan, J. A., Doering, R. W., & Bradley, S. J. (1983). Human figure drawings of gender-problem children: A comparison of sibling, psychiatric, and normal controls. *Journal of Abnormal Child Psychology, 11,* 287–298.